A SHORT TEXTBOOK OF
Psychiatry

For Non-Psychiatrists

RP Rajarethinam MD

About the Author:
Rajaprabhakaran Rajarethinam (RP) obtained his medical degree in Madurai Medical College, Madurai, India. He was trained in psychiatry at Madras Medical College, India. He further trained in University of Iowa and University of Michigan in the USA. He worked at Wayne State University, Detroit MI and McLean Hospital, Belmont, MA. He is in private practice in Ann Arbor, MI USA

He can be reached @rpmmc or rpmmc@yahoo.com and @rpraj on telegram

Author Disclosure:
The author has received research support from various pharmaceutical companies including Johnson and Johnson, Astra Zenica, Neurocrine, Allergan, Avanir, Pfizer, Boehringer Engelheim, and others

Copyright © Rajaprabhakaran Rajarethinam 2019

ISBN: 9781704283173

Typeset in Palatino from Adobe inDesign

Contents

1. Challenges in the Understanding of Mental Illnesses — 1
2. History of Psychiatry — 5
3. Psychology, Social Sciences, and Human Behavior — 11
4. Neuroscience — 16
5. Psychosis and Schizophrenia — 25
6. Mood Disorders — 35
7. Anxiety Disorders — 49
8. PTSD and Trauma Related Disorders — 69
9. Eating Disorders — 77
10. Alcoholism and Substance Use Disorders — 84
11. Personality Disorders — 102
12. Dissociative Disorders & Somatic Symptoms Disorders — 119
13. Dementia — 129
14. Child Psychiatry — 137
15. Sleep Disorders — 160
16. Sexual Disorders — 172
17. Psychopharmacology — 186
18. Psychotherapy — 208
19. Evaluation of a Patient with Mental Illness. — 214
20. Miscellaneous Topics — 220

To my wife

Acknowledgments

I am sincerely thankful to a number of people who inspired, supported, and helped me to complete this project. The social work staff from St. Mary's Hospital, Livonia MI inspired me to start this project. The nurses in McLean Hospital, Belmont MA essentially gave me the idea. The wonderful staff members at Huron Valley PACE experimented with the idea of 20 lectures turning into 20 chapters for a book, that gave me impetus. Dr. Mukundu Nagesh, (one of my most respected classmates), helped me with line by line review of the content language and style. Dr. Swaroop Thangam for his feedback in early drafts. Sankaralingam Arunkumar, of Icon Lifesciences, Chennai, a friend and relative, who graciously agreed to print and distribute this book. Kristen Willmer completed full editing. Alexa Sotiroff provided the diagrams. Zach Sila, Abigail Swanson, Elizabeth Einig and Alexa Sotiroff helped with editing and formatting. My wife and children, without whom I would not have ventured into this (may have done something better!).

Preface

A few years ago, I received a phone call from the hospital in the middle of the night. The caller, a new social worker, relayed a message from the ER doctors explaining that there was a "manic, psychotic and suicidal" patient. When I asked for more information about the patient, the caller was at a loss to explain what she meant by psychosis or mania. As this happened a few more times, the social workers, annoyed by my frequent questions, invited me to give a lecture in their monthly meeting. They wanted me to describe what I need precisely or what the social worker needs to know before presenting a case to me. Over the years as a clinician-educator, I have found it a joy to explain and teach students with various backgrounds about mental illnesses and the nuances of psychiatric symptoms and presentations. I happily obliged.

As it turned out, the aforementioned patient happened to be locked out of her home and wanted a place to stay overnight. While the decision to admit the patient was inevitable because she was convincing in her claim of suicidality. However, her claim of being manic and psychotic needed to be assessed appropriately. This assessment is not as difficult as one might imagine.

Another experience comes to my mind. On my first day on call as a psychiatry resident, I received a consult request from the orthopedics department. They were receiving a patient transferred from another VA facility, and the patient happened to have a diagnosis of schizophrenia. Before they even saw the patient, they called the psych on-call doctor for a consult. I answered the page and asked them why they needed a consult. The poor intern on the other end told me, "I don't know... The patient has schizophrenia. We don't know what to do with him. Is he going to be OK or jump out of the window...? Don't know. Just making sure he will be OK." I told them I would come and check on the patient when he reached the hospital. That evening, I walked into the patient's room and saw this young man, lying in bed with orthopedic casts all over his body, with both legs propped up with weights and pulleys. He was pleasantly smiling at me while all the doctors around him seemed to be too busy to greet me. I said, "I guess you may not need a consult" and walked away.

Experiences such as these are the inspiration for this book. The callers above may have had different reasons for not evaluating the patient, however, I believe that a bit of training and knowledge would help them handle such situations with more confidence. I believe that people who do not deal with mental illnesses regularly may benefit from a simple explanation of psychiatry.

It is also common for the patients to report a diagnosis instead of symptoms, which may be misleading. It is crucial for the clinician to ask appropriate questions to elicit and understand the presenting symptoms and reach an appropriate diagnosis. A clear diagnosis and understanding of the patient's symptoms are crucial for an appropriate intervention or treatment plan, especially in psychiatry, as there are no objective diagnostic tools like blood tests or X-Rays.

While a diagnosis of a mental illness itself is questionable under the best circumstances, misunderstanding of symptoms is quite common in the field. Frequently, the mood instability of a personality disorder is misunderstood and misidentified as bipolar illness, by patients and professionals alike. When I consult doctors from other specialties, I frequently find myself needing to explain the differences between symptoms that appear the same, but from different diagnoses (e.g., delirium vs. psychosis).

Inspiration for this book, which I hope provides some clarity to the psychiatric symptoms and diagnoses, comes from these encounters. Much of the content in this manuscript comes verbatim from these repeated explanations to my colleagues and patients. At least some of them, possibly trying to be polite, told me that the explanation helped them understand the illness better. I hope this book helps a few more.

I hope that this book will help my target audience, including nurses, social workers, and doctors from other specialties, understand better what we, as psychiatrists, mean when we say something. And, help them understand the intricacies of the psychiatric symptoms and their diagnostic implications in various clinical contexts so that they can provide appropriate care for those afflicted by mental illnesses.

Introduction

This book is written in a simple easy-to-read style using language that resembles bedside teaching - the best teaching in medicine. The target audience of this book include a variety of clinicians including, social workers, case managers and mental heath technicians, primary care physicians and physicians in other specialties. I hope this book will help improve people's understanding of what they are dealing with when they are helping patients with mental illness. My idea behind this book is to answer any questions a clinician who happens to see a patient with a mental illness might have. I have made an attempt to write this manuscript, imagining myself answering and explaining those questions. The length, emphasis and structure of each chapter and topic reflect the commonality of the clinical situations. If this book does not appear to be a conventional textbook, it is intentional.

Chapter 1

Challenges in the Understanding of Mental Illnesses

It is estimated that more than half of all human beings will endure a mental illness in their lifetime. If not us, someone we love will suffer from a behavioral problem at some point. Seldom life-threatening, mental illness and substance abuse cause immense suffering and are estimated to be the most significant cause of disability in the global burden of disease. Yet, very little is known about the science of normal and abnormal behavior, and our understanding of mental illnesses lags behind to our understanding of physical illnesses.

In general, the cause of mental illnesses is unknown, the mechanisms behind human behavior are not well understood, diagnosis is arbitrary, treatment is based on symptoms, the symptoms are subjective and overlap between diseases, there is rarely a cure, and even the distinction between normal and abnormal is frequently unclear. To complicate the issue further, the stigma and the negative attitude towards individuals with behavioral problems make psychiatry one of the least understood and least desired branches of medicine.

Diagnosing and treating a mental illness is very different from physical illnesses. The diagnosis is arbitrary, which some would argue that it is nothing more than a clinician's opinion of whatever the patient says. A patient may be biased by his or her personal beliefs, perception, experience, and knowledge when reporting symptoms. Psychiatric symptoms are often exaggerated (anxiety), minimized (drug use), or even denied (psychosis). The clinician may be influenced by his or her own set of bias[1], perception, or judgment over the patient. There is no hard

---

[1] The mental anguish of a slave including his or her desire to escape slavery was described as a mental condition by an American Physician Samuel Cartwright in 1851 who surmised that blacks by nature would want to be slaves and if someone is not comfortable with being a slave, they must be mentally ill.

evidence: no blood test, scan or a bacterium and so the diagnosis cannot be proved or disproved. The lack of evidence-based diagnosis leads to extreme variability in the assessment of an individual with behavioral problems.

For example, what if a successful businessman at the end of a busy season, feels "depressed and bored to death" because there is nothing to do? What if someone lost their spouse of 30 years and feels depressed to the point of killing themselves? They both could be diagnosed with depression, or just explained away as circumstantial or understandable. What if the businessman insists on taking medication and the widower refuses help despite being severely depressed and suicidal?[2] As a clinician, both cases may present a dilemma about how to make an appropriate clinical decision.

The clinician constantly faces such dilemmas and challenges. Sometimes, it feels unfair to characterize a stressful life event as a disease and intervene, but, at the same time, it is also unfair to ignore someone's suffering. An unambiguous characterization of the illness and a standardization with a valid and reliable diagnosis is necessary for the clinicians to operate under or get paid (Insurances do not pay without a diagnosis, or sometimes even with diagnoses such as personality disorders or substance abuse. By the way, no one pays for an annual mental check-up!). At the same time, overdiagnosis may lead to false positives, and underdiagnosis or minimization may deny appropriate care and support for the suffering.

The dangers of diagnosis without proof can be problematic. Homosexuality was considered a disease by DSM until 1973, which may have led some to believe that they are mentally ill due to their sexual orientation. In the 1950s schizophrenia was overdiagnosed in minorities in the USA. Even now, ADHD is estimated to be prevalent at 5% in the USA and 1% in the UK due to the differences in criteria used. Some areas in the USA, parental reports show a lot more than 5% of the children are diagnosed with ADHD.

However, every single day, we, psychiatrists and therapists indulge in diagnosing people without proof, treat them with powerful medications, call ourselves experts, and get paid! Yet, the diagnostic criteria, as employed by the DSM and ICD, are critical and important advances in mental illness and medicine in general. Although some critics may disagree with the use of criteria, calling it "cookbook medicine," there

---

[2] Mourning used to be an exemption in the diagnosis of depression. DSM 5 took the "mourning exception" meaning if a person in mourning continues to be depressed after two weeks, they can be diagnosed with depression the disease.

is no better system to identify the sufferings of several billion people in order to help them. It will be chaos without these criteria.

Standardization is important in all walks of medicine, from diagnosing hypertension to staging cancer. Without a good understanding of the type and stage of cancer, we cannot offer clear diagnostic, therapeutic, or prognostic estimates. We cannot compare patients or treatment options or communicate with each other. We cannot conduct research and generalize the results. Every single aspect of medicine, from surgeries to vaccination or palliative care, needs criteria to measure symptoms and treat appropriately.

Adding confusion to the struggle of standardization of psychiatric diagnoses, the symptoms transcend across diagnoses. Patients with depression frequently have anxiety and vice versa. Psychosis can happen in mania and depression. Anxiety and depression can cooccur in schizophrenia and bipolar illness. In addition, comorbidity or co-occurring diagnoses can also confuse the presentation. Patients with one mental illness seem to be susceptible to others, especially alcohol and substance use. While we emphasize so much on the diagnosis and its specificity for consistent treatment, most of the treatment in psychiatry is, in fact, symptomatic; meaning, no matter how you get a certain symptom, the treatment is the same. For example, psychosis, whether it is from schizophrenia, mania, depression, or organic causes such as Parkinson's disease, or even due to drugs, is treated with the same medications. In spite of this, interestingly, medications are typically tested and approved based on the diagnosis.

Sometimes, the same medications work for different conditions. For example, antidepressants are the treatment of choice for anxiety disorders. Mania (with or without psychosis) is treated with antipsychotics and many antipsychotics and mood stabilizers help augment the treatment of depression. However, mood stabilizers do not work for mood swings caused by a personality disorder.

Stigma and attitude influence the approach and treatment greatly. Behavioral problems are often seen as something under the control of the individual. For example, no one would blame a person with paralysis or a fracture for not running, but we easily blame someone who refuses to do something because of anxiety, for not trying hard enough. We tend to suspect the person with any abnormal behavior as wanton, intentional or resulting from poor self-control. This attitude adds to the stigma and bias, which in turn, may influence our willingness to help them.

Behavior that is deviant, abnormal, or even slightly non-conforming, impacts others, and so, the instigator of such behavior is typically sanctioned or subjected to reprimand. Some behaviors such as violence, even when instigated without someone's control, elicit scorn from others - not sympathy. Assessing an abnormal behavior as an illness can be very easy in some cases like psychosis but difficult in others such as alcoholism or anxiety. In addition, patients with behavioral problems evoke a strong emotional response from clinicians, be it sympathy, scorn, ridicule or disdain, influencing the clinician's attitude and behavior.

All these issues affect the day to day life of mental health clinicians, as well as the lives of those seeking help from them. One wonders endlessly how these clinicians keep a straight face and do their best to help the patients. This is an example of excellence in the face of adversity.

Yet, there is great hope. Advances in the understanding of the brain, behavior, and psychopharmacology have made a tremendous impact on millions of people so far. Imagine the plight of severely mentally ill patients centuries ago. We have come a long way from unshackling our patients from the dungeons and asylums to accepting them and living with them side by side. But there is still a long way to go. There is so much suffering by billions of people, both obvious and untold. I sincerely hope that this book will help educate and inform clinicians towards a better understanding of mental illnesses so that they can provide better care, and, I sincerely hope that this book will take us forward, even if it is a small step.

Chapter 2

History of Psychiatry

The Vedas, a series of ancient Indian texts on philosophy and medicine that dates back to about 1,000 – 3,000 BC, describe mental illnesses similar to schizophrenia, paranoia, and bipolar disorder. They attribute these behavioral deviations to Divine Curses, a belief still adhered to by some in India. Similar ideas of demonic possession, evil eye, or sorcery were commonly held across most ancient cultures trying to explain thought, speech, and behavior that defy logic. Babylonians, Mesopotamians, Assyrians, and the ancient Greeks shared this attribution of demonic possession to abnormal behavior. Ancient Egyptians believed that madness could result from gastrointestinal irregularity!

In the golden age of Athens, around 400-600 BC, the Greek "naturalized" mental illness alongside their advances in other domains of reason. They moved away from the idea of the Gods and supernatural powers influencing thought and action to individuals, thus humanizing the normal and abnormal behavior. Hippocrates, the father of medicine (460 BC to 370 BC), wrote about epilepsy "the sacred disease appears to me to be no more divine nor more sacred than other diseases... Men regard this as divine because of ignorance and wonder as this disease is unlike others...". Along with other physicians of his time, he proposed that all illnesses may result from disturbances of internal bodily fluids, such as bile, a theory known as humorism. Melancholy, depicting severe depression, literally means black bile (melano is black and chole is bile) in Greek. This thinking was followed and propagated by Galen, another Greek physician, who would greatly influence medicine, including mental illness, and medical education, for the next millennium.

When Christianity was introduced into the Roman Empire in AD 313, the emphasis on reason as the essence of human behavior was changed to thoughts centered around faith, sins, redemption, and divine will. Good and evil were reasoned to be the handiwork of God and the Devil and their struggle inside a human mind. This thinking continued until at least the 18th century when "reason" once again became the core of European thinking regarding mental illness. Unfortunately, the belief in demonic possession and the attribution of mental illness to witches led to widespread barbaric witch-hunting in the 14th and 15th centuries. 200,000 individuals, mostly women, may have been tortured and executed.

Around this time, Shakespeare (1564-1616) incorporated mental illness in his writings to enrich many of his characters including King Lear's madness, Jaques' melancholy, Macbeth's visions, Lady Macbeth's sleepwalking and the obsessions of Leontes. He also wrote in Macbeth about alcohol and sex "it provoketh the desire but taketh away the performance." Robert Burton (1577-1640) a contemporary of Shakespeare published "The Anatomy of Melancholy" which is considered a classic work of English literature, although written as a medical text. It is believed that he suffered from depression and professed in his book that "I write of melancholy, by being busy to avoid melancholy. There is no greater cause of melancholy than idleness, no better cure than business." He apparently rewrote the book several times, suggesting that the poor Oxford scholar had multiple relapses.

Rene Descartes (1596-1650), considered as the father of modern philosophy, introduced the idea that consciousness is a component of the body (famously credited for "cogito ergo sum" meaning "I think, therefore I am"). William Pargeter (1760-1810), a physician, expanded upon Descartes' thinking of reason as the basis of humans and their consciousness.

The treatment of abnormal behavior followed the beliefs of the times and the interventions typically included efforts to drive the evil force from the bodies. This resulted in torture and killings of the purportedly possessed. However, there is archaeological evidence of ancient human skulls being trephined (a hole was drilled), which is believed to be an attempted treatment for mental illness, suggesting the possibility that some looked for evidence inside the skull for unusual behavior. As time went by, individuals with behavioral and emotional problems were sequestered in asylums, the earliest of which were built in Iraq and Europe, with the intention of protecting the society from the "mad."

The Birth of Asylums

Traditionally, families took care of the mentally ill, whether they were docile and manageable or violent needing restraints. Mostly, they were tied down in dungeons or left in the street to beg. Formal segregation started towards the end of Middle Ages in Europe, partly influenced by Christian belief in charity. In London, the religious house of St. Mary of Bethlehem (known as Bedlam) was founded in 1247 and became a popular place for housing the mentally ill. Bedlam still functions as a fine institute for mental health care and research in South London, as part of the NHS. Soon, asylums were built around Europe to house the mentally ill, mostly for convenience, safety, or legal reasons, rather than for treatment. The treatment or management of the mentally ill in these asylums mostly consisted of various forms of restraints such as straitjackets and chains. A visitor to these asylums would certainly be appalled by the treatment of fellow human beings.

Jean-Baptiste Pussin (1745-1811) a superintendent at Bicêtre hospital, banned less than humane treatment, such as restraints, and engaged in talking and listening to the patients. Philippe Pinel (1745-1026), a colleague of Pussin, used the same approach in Salpêtrière and popularized "Moral Therapy" - an idea of treating patients with psychological means to change the "psyche" by listening and talking to them. A similar change was instituted by William Tuke in England and Vicenzo Chiarugi in Italy. They believed in biological interventions and emphasized the concept of disease. The late-1700s and the 19th century saw an explosion of the number of asylums along with the increase in state oversight and regulations. The approach of the asylums changed from "'safety for the society" to "safe and humane'" treatment of the mentally ill. Psychiatry as a diagnostic and therapeutic medical science established its roots around this time.

Mental Illness and the Brain

The emphasis on the brain as the seat of mental illness started with Thomas Willis (1621-75) coining the term neurology for the science of the brain and the nervous system. He believed that specific areas of the brain were responsible for mental illnesses. William Cullen (The University of Birmingham, mid-1700s) in an attempt to classify diseases, grouped disease of the nervous system as "neuroses" (although the word neurosis took a completely different meaning in the post-Freudian era). Inspired by Lockean philosophy of empiricism that emphasized experience and evidence as opposed to blind faith, Thomas Arnold and others (the late 1700s) argued that human behavior and its abnormalities should be studied with observation and experimentation. Pinel's psychological approach and Chiarugi's disease concept also fueled this approach. These developments led to the proposed distinctions of different maladies based on the mind and its functions.

As a direct result of the "asylum movement," where patients were housed for years, a systematic observation and data collection became possible. Jean-Etienne Esquirol, a student of Pinel, wrote the classic textbook "Mental Maladies, A treatise on insanity" in 1845. He distinguished epilepsy from mental illnesses and pioneered exclusive hospitals for patients with epilepsy. At the same time, the study of neurology and the investigation of the nervous system by postmortem dissection gained popularity. Although spirochetes were not discovered as the cause of syphilis during this time, Antoine Laurent Bayle (1799-1858), a French physician, described "general paralysis of insane" (GPI – is a syphilitic brain infection that can lead to various behavioral problems). He demonstrated brain abnormalities as possible cause for this "insanity" by postmortem dissection.

Around the same time, Guillaume Duchenne (1806-1875), described tabes dorsalis or syphilitic myelopathy, which established that the origins of mental and behavioral abnormalities can be traced to the brain. His contemporary, sometimes dubbed as the Napoleon of the neuroses Jean-Martin Charcot (1825-1893), a famous clinical professor of the nervous system at the Salpêtrière, was convinced that a neurological basis could be found for a range of illnesses, from migraines and seizures to hallucinations and depression. His lectures introduced orderly thinking of the neurological and psychiatric illnesses and influenced many of his famous students including Freud, Babinski, Tourette, and Binet. While Charcot made significant discoveries in neurological disorders, he did not make much progress in mental illness despite his conviction. He studied hypnotism and animal magnetism, the best available "technologies" of his time to study the mind.

Germany had a different tradition of university-based research. Carl Wernicke (1848-1905) studied localization of brain functions. He located the speech areas in the brain and wrote an authoritative three-volume manual of brain diseases (1883). Around this time in Germany, Franz Joseph Gall (1758-1828) introduced Phrenology, a (pseudo)science of studying mental faculties based on the bumps and shapes of the skull. He tried to prove racial differences based on this. While reviled by many as unscientific, this became very popular, and, unfortunately, encouraged stereotypical thinking and racism.

Another line of thinking, partly influenced by Darwinian thoughts of evolution and the notion of survival of the fittest, known as "degenerationism," also took hold among some. Benedict Morel (1809-1873) wrote that degeneration might happen over generations starting from "imbecility" and moving towards sterility, "proving" the extinction of the unfit. Magnus Huss in Sweden proposed alcoholism as a concept and claimed that it was a model of degeneration of the physical and moral self. It became convenient to blame such a degeneration to alcoholism, criminality, poverty, and mental illness, all of which co-occur. Cesare Lombroso (1836-1909) went further and associated such degeneration to physical stigmata and conveniently denigrated non-European races based on this thinking. Sexual deviances and homosexuality were also believed to result from moral degeneration. In the USA, George Beard popularized the term "Neurasthenia" - a nervous breakdown which he claimed resulted from the immoral aspirations of the materialistic world. The assassination of US President Garfield (1881) and the ensuing trial of Charles Guiteau, strengthened the psychiatrists' belief that "moral degeneration" was the cause of such heinous acts. In the US, this belief led to some Eugenic methods of confining and sterilizing "degenerates" long before Nazi Germany. The eugenic movement also influenced restrictive US immigration policy that prohibited the immigration of the mentally ill, along with non-whites.

20th-Century Psychiatry

Around the turn of the 20th century, a number of major conceptual advances happened in psychiatry along with parallel advances in the other walks of medicine. Progressive psychiatrists of the time tried to understand mental illnesses by applying the ideas from evolutionary biology, microbiological theory, and electrophysiology. Some of them saw mesmerism and spiritualism as intellectual embarrassments rather than scientific methods. Henry Maudsley, John Hughlings Jackson, and Herbert Spencer (and Sigmund Freud) were among the proponents of applying Darwinian evolutionism to the science of behavior and mental illness. But it was Emil Kraepelin (1856-1926) who made the innovative breakthrough of his time for which, some consider him as the father of modern psychiatry.

Kraepelin introduced nosology and classification to mental illness with an emphasis on the longitudinal course and long-term disability or deterioration as opposed to the current psychological state. Observing patients through their lifetime, Kraepelin differentiated schizophrenia from bipolar illness. He coined the term "Dementia Praecox" expanding the idea of Morel who described "demence precoce" in describing schizophrenia. He also included Karl Kahlbaum's description of catatonia and Ewald Hecker's description of "hebephrenia" in this condition that later became schizophrenia. Specifically, he differentiated dementia praecox from the "circular insanity" described by Fahlret - which he called as manic-depressive psychoses. He observed that manic-depressive psychoses did not go through the deterioration found in dementia praecox. Although doubts continue to exist about the separation of these diagnoses, this was a major advance in the science of mental illness and Kraepelinian thinking still influences the classification to this day.

The word schizophrenia was coined by Eugen Bleuler (1857-1939), a Swiss psychiatrist. With his astute clinical observations, he broke away from the existing concepts of dementia praecox (or early-onset dementia) and the dogmatic Freudian thinking of subconscious and the unknown. He proclaimed that schizophrenia results from a split of mental faculties (this "split" is commonly misunderstood as a split in personality). He proposed that there are four fundamental abnormalities in schizophrenia: 1) associational disturbances, 2) ambivalence, 3) affective disturbances and 4) autism. Here, autism means that the patient "lives with himself" or has impaired interpersonal interaction. These are known as Bleuler's four "As." He believed that schizophrenia could range in severity and the "dementia," or the cognitive deficits, were just components of the illness.

For a period after World War II, psychoanalysis took hold of psychiatry and understanding of the mental illnesses in some parts of the world. Later in the 20th century, however, the science advanced and as medications such as chlorpromazine and tricyclic antidepressants were introduced, and the thinking became more scientific. Categorization and classification of the behavioral problems improved and gained reliability and validity through scientific methods.

Along with the development of psychoanalysis, advances in psychology and theories of personality development, psychiatry advanced in the 20th century in an unprecedented manner. The understanding of normal and abnormal behavior moved long ways from the idea of divine intervention. Application of scientific methodology, objective studies, and replicable experiments contributed to this advancement. Statistics and advances in epidemiology enabled the development of better classification of the mental illness. Discoveries from neuroscience contribute to the steady improvement in our understanding of behavior. While psychiatry is still considered, sometimes derisively, as the art form of the medicine (that lacks science), advances in science and technology, will bring mental health to on par with the rest of the medicine sooner or later.

Chapter 3

Psychology, Social Sciences, and Human Behavior

Psychology is a vast social science focused on human mental functions and behavior. It is beyond the scope of this book to provide an introduction to psychology. In this chapter, I will discuss the aspects of psychology that are relevant to the practice of psychiatry.

Learning Theory

Learning is an acquired change in behavior (or skill) resulting from experience and not from an innate ability. Throughout our lives, we constantly learn new things that influence and change our behavior, attitudes, and interests. Learning plays a major role in mental illnesses such as anxiety, depression, and others. Understanding the basics of learning theory would not only help understand the behavior and development of symptoms, but it will also aid in the treatment.

The fundamentals of learning theory come from Ivan Pavlov's famous dog that salivated for the bell ring. Pavlov, while researching the digestive system of the dogs, noticed them salivating when the dog handler who brings food walked in, even if they were not given the meat. He suspected that the dogs "learn" to expect food with certain cues, like the handler walking in. He designed an experiment where he provided food after ringing a bell. In due course, the dogs would salivate for the bell ringing even when there was no food. Thus, he trained or "conditioned" the dog to salivate for the bell after several pairings of the bell with food (powdered meat in this case). The bell ringing in this context is called the "conditioned stimulus," and the salivation for the bell is called "conditioned response." We all remember a certain cologne or a song that reminds us of our middle school teacher, first love or an unpleasant event. This process is called classical conditioning.

Operant conditioning, on the other hand, pertains to the behavior changes that happen as a consequence of our actions, rather than our response to a stimulus. In other words, operant conditioning is any learning that happens as a result of rewards and punishments for our actions. A typical lab example is a cat locked in a box, who learns to get out by pressing a lever that opens the door. They may initially do it accidentally or randomly, but they soon learn to do it as the result is rewarding. Similarly, they may also learn to do a specific thing like pressing a lever to avoid electric shock (punishment avoidance). In these examples, the behavior is shaped, strengthened, or weakened by rewards and punishments.

This type of learning is involved in social learning and behavioral change. We do learn and modify our behavior on a day-to-day basis using operant conditioning techniques that include punishments and rewards. Behaviorism is a field of study that focuses on how learning changes our behavior. John B Watson and, later, B.F. Skinner popularized behaviorism and expanded it into almost all aspects of human behavior, including individual and group behaviors.

Principles of learning theory are used successfully in the day-to-day management of patients with mental illnesses and employed when behavioral changes are needed for the wellbeing of the patient, such as diet and exercise. Cognitive-behavioral therapies (CBT) help people suffering from depression, OCD, personality disorders, and others. One simple example of CBT is exposure therapy for phobia (e.g., fear of flying), where patients are exposed to the condition that causes the fear (flying) repeatedly to a point they eventually lose their fear. The learning (or unlearning) can be a powerful tool in managing various psychiatric symptoms. Of the many psychotherapeutic techniques, CBT and variants have been scientifically proven to be effective, sometimes as effective or even superior to medications.

Human Development

The biological aspects of human development and the maturation of the brain are discussed elsewhere. It is important to remember that the brain, like the rest of the body, goes through a significant amount of growth and maturation, which corresponds to our psychological, and intellectual development. Jean Piaget (1896-1980), a Swiss psychologist who studied children and their development of thought process, described human development into four stages:

1) Sensorimotor Stage (from birth to 2 years of age): In this age, babies explore the world around them by their five sensory modes and develop control of their motor function. They do not perceive anything

other than their immediate surroundings and develop "object permanence," meaning they learn to understand the existence of an object, even when it is hidden from view.

2) Pre-operational Stage (age 2 to about age 7): Children develop language and understand its meanings. While they do not yet understand logic or morals, they understand good and bad. Their concepts and ideas are primitive and still egocentric, meaning they have difficulty looking at things from others' point of view. They use imagination and understand cause and effect as proximal rather than logical (occurring together vs. cause and effect), and their logic is simple and primitive. At this age, they ask a lot of questions that start with "why" and struggle to understand causation.

3) Concrete Operational Stage (age 7 to age 11): They develop logic and reasoning, although still rigid in their thinking. They can see through conceptual similarities and differences (such as edible fruits or mammals). They may start to think more like adults, but they are still not good at abstract thinking or understanding hypotheses. They master the idea of cause and effect and understand "reversibility" – an idea that objects and numbers can be changed and reversed (demonstrated by pouring a glass of milk in a cup and back into a bottle or borrowing money).

4) Formal Operational Stage (age 11 to 18 and beyond): In this age, teens develop abstract thinking, deductive reasoning, and the ability to understand subtleties of various concepts. They are able to reason, contemplate different aspects or points of view, and make independent decisions. Such abstract thinking leads to a curiosity over diverse topics such as religion, and philosophy. This coincides with the hormonal changes as well as rapid development and maturation of the brain and body. They form self-identity, develop strong likes and dislikes, and try to reach or take a definitive stand on everything. While they are extremely flexible in their thinking, they see others, especially authority figures, in a more critical manner.

Healthy psychological development is essential to become a well-functioning adult. Physical, emotional or sexual abuse or neglect in crucial stages correlate with psychopathology later in life.

Psychoanalysis

Sigmund Freud, a neurologist by training, was inspired by the use of hypnotism and mesmerism while working under Charcot and developed psychoanalysis as a new therapeutic technique to treat mental illnesses. He also proposed new theories of psychological construct and the development of personality, which supported and explained his method of intervention: psychoanalysis. He believed that during the developmental stage, children and even infants, suppress uncomfortable thoughts by a process he called "repression." He claimed that these suppressed thoughts stay at a level below conscious awareness, which he called the "unconscious." He concluded that such undesirable, repressed thoughts lead to internal conflicts, which in turn cause psychopathology later in life.

As they are purportedly "unconscious" and "uncomfortable," these thoughts and conflicts, he believed, would not be freely expressed by patients. So, he devised a technique called "free association" in which the patient is encouraged to talk without inhibition or restraint. A trained psychoanalyst would listen to these, interpret them, and discover the hidden conflicts. He also resorted to interpreting dreams for meanings and clues of the supposedly hidden, internal conflicts. Freud famously proposed the "Oedipus Complex" in which he believed all conflicts are the result of the latent sexuality of the developing age, which "sexualized" entire psychopathology, according to some critics.

Freud believed that the human mind is constructed into three parts: the id, ego, and superego. The id being the primal force within, that operates with unchecked, and unconscious desire, the ego being the conscious self that is based in reality, and the superego being the force behind moral principles of the psyche. This theoretical construct helped him explain the therapeutic resolution and symptomatic improvement, which he believed happened after psychoanalysis.

He believed that the psychopathology results from suppressed desires (libido) during psycho-sexual development, and psychoanalysis brings these to the surface and resolves psychopathology. He considered the patient's reaction towards the analyst as "transference," which he claimed depends upon the nature of the repressed conflict and the development of the individual with that conflict. Understanding transference, he believed, is a major component of patient's improvement.

These are theoretical proposals or hypotheses that cannot be verified objectively. This led to widespread criticism, which was sometimes aggressive, vehement and vitriolic. Karl Popper criticized Freud's theories as unscientific as they are "unfalsifiable," meaning, an experiment capable of disproving these theories cannot be designed or conducted and, thus do not meet the basic tenets of science. Hans Eysenck famously quoted that Freud set back the study and science of psychology by about 50 years. There are some who "wish Freud was not born" and say that psychoanalysis was the most successful pseudoscience. Eugen Bleuler, upon resigning from the International Psychoanalytic Society, wrote that "... such dogmatic, all or nothing ideas are fit only for religion or politics but not science."

While there is severe criticism of psychoanalysis from "biologically minded" psychiatrists on one end, and an implicit acceptance without any belief in the middle, there is also ardent support and following among many psychiatrists, psychologists and patients. Many among the believers contend that this is more of an art form and a theoretical concept that is helpful for patients, and, so, the objectivity and the scientific validity may not matter.

However, the practical or impractical nature of psychoanalysis, which requires weekly sessions for years, has made the practice less viable and unpopular. Not only is psychoanalysis a luxury in terms of time and money, but the requirement of intellectual and psychological sophistication limited its reach to the rich and worried well. The severely mentally ill and elderly were deemed unanalyzable. The advent of modern medications such as SSRIs to treat anxiety and depression have also made long and arduous therapy less desirable (Prozac cured psychoanalysis!).

Chapter 4

Neuroscience

The Brain

It is widely believed that the human brain is the most complex structure in the universe, assuming there are no other more intelligent creatures with more complex brains out there. Studying such an advanced organ poses a number of challenges. Although biologically similar, animal brains cannot be subject to experiments that mimic human functions as they do not seem to indulge in human things like reading, calculation, or gossip[1]. While there are ethical reasons not to conduct invasive experimental research on human brains, there are no perfect tools, invasive or noninvasive, to "look into one's brain" while it is doing complex mental tasks. Besides the lesion studies, meaning, looking at how damage in the brain relates to functional loss, there are no foolproof tools to study cognition. However, the field of neuroscience is advancing leaps and bounds. The prospects of better understanding the brain are enormous. Better knowledge of the brain will help us not only understand normal and abnormal behavior but also may lead to happiness and peace for humanity with endless possibilities in the resolution of conflicts amongst humans, personal to international.

The Neuron

The building block of the brain is the neuron. While it may be obvious, it is interesting to look at the way a neuron is built and consider it in the context of what it does. The figure below shows muscle tissue that contracts unidirectionally, heart muscle that needs to contract together, and a neuron that predominantly shows connections. The main function of neurons, as you can imagine, is to convey messages from one cell to

---

[1] Although, there are some recent reports that monkeys, dolphins, and whales communicate with others and gossip, even about the ogling humans. I wonder what they talk about us.

another (neuronal or other), through long axons that can be several feet long or short, microscopic dendrites. The messages are transmitted via electrical impulses or complex biochemical signals. At the basic level, a message or a signal can turn something on or off, but at a complex level, these transmissions enable a variety of brain functions from hunger and

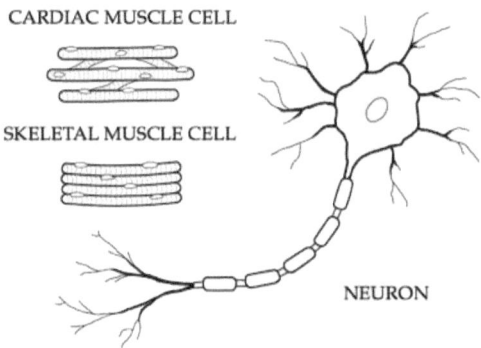

sex to philosophical introspection about the meaning of life. Our brains have about 100 billion neurons, and each one may have up to 200,000 dendrites or connections. These help the neurons to form circuits ranging from a simple loop that helps us withdraw from pain, reflexively, to understanding, or pretending to understand, the stock market. One can imagine the number of permutations and combinations possible in processing signals or information. It is estimated that the brain makes about one million new connections each second, based upon internal and external experiences of the individual, thus making each brain a unique organ. For better or worse, you are making a few odd connections while reading this!

The Synapse

A synapse is a junction where a neuron passes a signal to another neuron or an end-organ, such as muscle (see figure below). A synapse may not just pass the information but modify it in many ways enabling the complex modulation of the brain circuits. The synapse becomes very complex with various neurochemicals traversing in and out, along with electrical responses. It is the presence and modulation of these neurochemicals that make us do things from throwing a ball to understanding Einstein's theories, and from enjoying alcohol to feeling love. Problems in this modulation of synaptic activity may lead to abnormal behavior, but it also provides an opportunity to manipulate the signals to treat an illness such as depression.

The Nervous System

Vertebrate animals have a nervous system that is divided into central

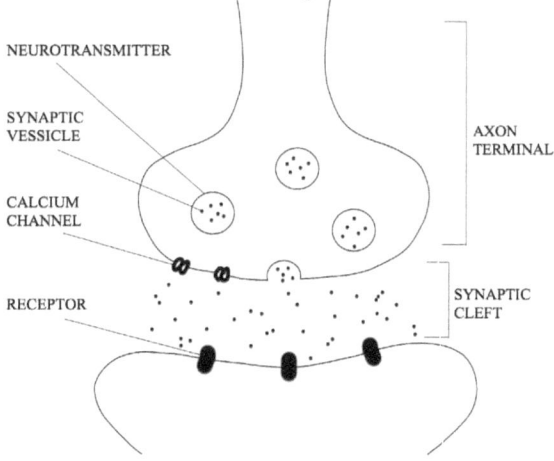

and peripheral nervous systems. The central nervous system consists of the brain and spinal cord, and the peripheral nervous system consists of nerves and the autonomic nervous system. Sensory nerves carry sensory information to the brain, such as light from the retina or pain from the foot, and the motor nerves carry the orders from the brain to the muscles. The autonomic nervous system controls involuntary functions such as involuntary breathing and heart rate. The brain is highly connected and controls everything about our body and mind. Many of the "higher" functions such as fear and anxiety affect the "lower" functions, like heart rate, muscle tension, and the bowels.

The brain weighs about 1.4 kilograms (three pounds), fills about 1300CC (44 ounces) and consists of neurons, their interconnections and support cells called glia. It floats in cerebrospinal fluid, which functions as a vibration dampener, cleaning system, and a moat that protects the brain against invasive elements. In spite of being housed in the hard shell of the skull, and separated from the rest of the body, the brain is often vulnerable to injuries and infections. The brain is divided into grey and white matter. Grey matter consists of the cell bodies of neurons, and the white matter consists of the axons and dendrites, sometimes referred together as "dendrils." The glia, or glial cells, which outnumber the neurons by 10:1, were originally believed to be support cells, but they are now believed to help neurons amplify the signals and are suspected of having a role in mental functions.

The brain structure, function, and connections are influenced and shaped mostly by genes and partly by the environment and experience.

The brain grows in spurts with expansion and pruning, starting at its largest (in relation to the body size) at the time of birth. As babies grow and learn, the brain accumulates new connections at a fast pace and increases in size, but it loses some volume in late teens due to the pruning of some connections, making the brain more efficient. It appears that the brain "settles down" in the adult form by age 25[2], although most of the development happens before age 18. While it is widely known that the brain constantly makes new connections all through life, it was believed, until recently, that new neuronal cells were never formed after birth. However, recent studies have shown that neurogenesis (formation of new neurons) happens all through life, albeit in a limited fashion, giving hope to the sufferers of "permanent" injuries such as paraplegia.

This growth or development of the brain seems to have major implications in mental illness. It is believed that many illnesses result from the abnormalities in the maturation or the development of the brain. In addition to influencing the basic structure of the brain, genes seem to influence how the brain develops and matures into the adult form, with the environment playing a smaller but significant role. In addition, environmental factors ranging from chemical exposure to psychological events can alter the gene expression by turning them on or off, thus influencing the brain. This phenomenon, which illustrates the gene environment-interaction is called epigenetics and has been an area of interest in mental health research in recent years.

Neuroimaging studies have shown that the total brain size (volume) increases from birth to the early teens, and then reduces in size, possibly due to the pruning of excess connections as the brain becomes more efficient. Dr. Jay Giedd at the NIMH child psychiatry branch has studied this extensively and reported that girls' brains peak in size at about 10.5 years of age and boys at 14.5 years of age. They also report that the white matter, which consists of axons and dendrites, continue to increase, but the grey matter follows a U-shaped growth pattern with an early maturation in sensory-motor areas, and later (late teens), maturation in the cognitively higher areas such as prefrontal cortex (decision making), inferior parietal lobe, and superior temporal gyrus (thinking and focus). There is a significant sex difference in the brain and there is also a significant difference in the maturation path of boys' and girls' brains.

---

2 It seems that we do not fully become adults or grown-ups until age 25 as far as the brain is considered. The insurance companies seem to have figured this out and so charge us a premium if we want to drive before age 25.

The Cortex

The cortex is arbitrarily divided into four lobes. The front of the brain, or the frontal lobe is situated right behind the forehead and ends at the central sulcus, a deep furrow that divides the frontal lobe from the parietal lobe. The frontal lobe is the biggest in humans, and the prefrontal area is believed to be responsible for executive functions and decision making. The gray matter right behind the frontal lobe is known as the parietal lobe, and the cortex at the back of the brain is called the occipital lobe. The temporal lobe is situated on the side above the ears. It is also more advanced in humans and it is believed to be responsible for language, emotion, attention, and associative learning and comprehension. The lateral sulcus is a major sulcus that runs horizontally and divides the temporal lobe below and the parietal lobe above. The parietal lobe consists of sensory processing areas and association areas, with verbal processing on the left side and visual-spatial processing on the right side. The occipital cortex processes visual information.

The frontal lobe consists of the motor cortex, premotor cortex, and related association cortices that are responsible for muscle contraction and movements. The connections between the thalamus and the frontal cortex are important in behavior. Lesions to magnocellular (the inner part of the thalamus) to orbital and medial cortex connections cause disinhibition, euphoria, and hyperkinesis. Disruption of the parvocellular (the outer layers of the thalamus) to dorsal and lateral prefrontal lobe connections result in apathy, cognitive impairment, hypokinesis, and psychomotor retardation. They may also play a role in attention, the ability to think in abstract and motor perseveration. Witzelsucht is a strange condition characterized by an inability to laugh at puns and jokes, particularly social ones, resulting from frontal lobe damage.

The temporal lobe has language association areas and Wernicke's area, which is responsible for receptive language (comprehension). Temporal lobe epilepsy or psychomotor seizures (sometimes called complex partial seizures) present with episodic symptoms of hallucinations and delusions. Lesions of the right parietal lobe lead to "denial and neglect" of the illness, which is called anosognosia. Famous cases include men with a right parietal lesion not shaving the left (opposite) side of the face. In addition, patients with a right-sided stroke often do not "worry" about the stroke; they may be aware of the stroke but behave as if it does not belong to them. A lesion in the dominant (left) parietal lobe results in right-left disorientation, agraphia, and acalculia is known as Gerstmann syndrome.

Occipital cortex is responsible for primary sensory processing of visual stimuli and holds visual associative cortex. Anton's syndrome is a rare condition resulting from bilateral blockade of posterior cerebral arteries leading to a stroke of the occipital area, causing "cortical blindness" in which, the eyes may see, but the brain does not sense or comprehend the vision.

The Inner Brain

The inner or core of the brain is phylogenetically older (evolved a lot earlier than the cortex) and these structures are involved in some of the basic functions essential for life.

The limbic system is not anatomically distinct and includes cortical areas such as limbic lobe, orbitofrontal cortex, piriform cortex, entorhinal area, and subcortical areas including hippocampus, amygdala, fornix, nucleus accumbens, hypothalamus, mamillary bodies, septal nuclei, and anterior nuclei of the thalamus. It is responsible for the control of mood, behavior, memory, and olfaction.

The thalamus is a round mass of grey matter inside the cerebrum which acts as a switchboard for all the sensory information from the body except olfaction (smell). Neurons carrying sensory information synapse here before being distributed to the cortex.

The hypothalamus is situated below the thalamus and is involved in a range of vital functions including hunger, thirst, emotion, and sleep. It is also involved in homeostasis - meaning balancing the body chemistry and the sleep-wake cycle. It controls the pituitary and is in the central loop of emotion control, and so, is an area of interest in emotional disorders such as depression.

The amygdala and hippocampus are situated close together deep in the temporal lobe. The hippocampus is responsible for making memories and is believed to be a key structure in ultra-short-term memory such as "holding" or remembering a phone number in your head before you dial it. The amygdala plays a significant role in the integration of emotions such as fear. The amygdala seems to tag memories with an emotion such as anxiety or fear, and thus an area of interest in anxiety disorders, phobia, and PTSD.

The brain stem is considered as the reptilian part of the brain as it is phylogenetically the oldest and simplest region, resembling the brains of reptiles. This area is responsible for basic functions such as breathing, heartbeat, and blood pressure. It is divided into the midbrain (helps with voluntary muscle movements), the pons (involved in sleep, level of consciousness, motor control and sensory integration) and the medulla or medulla oblongata is the tail end of the brain where it continues down as the spinal cord. The medulla plays a role in heart rate and breathing. The bulk of the medulla is white matter fibers traversing up into the brain.

The cerebellum is the small globe-like structure behind the brain and is involved in posture, balance, and movement. Alcohol affects the cerebellum and causes swaying while inebriated. There is evidence for cerebellum's role in thought and behavior.

Neurotransmitters

Neurotransmitters are chemicals produced by the body and secreted into the neuronal synapse. They are typically produced and stored in small globules called synaptic vesicles in the axon terminal (presynapse) and are released when an electrical or biochemical signal reaches the axon terminal. Once released into the synaptic junction, they bind with the receptors in the post-synaptic neuron to activate (or inhibit) the signal downstream, resulting in "synaptic transmission." The neurotransmitters are available in the junction for a very short period of time before they are deactivated by either a reuptake from the releasing axon or through enzymatic degradation in the synapse. The presence and attachment of the neurotransmitter to the receptor may initiate a cascade of events in the receiving neuron (or a non-neuronal cell like a muscle or a gland).

This system enables us to manipulate the brain with exogenous chemicals from alcohol to street drugs as well as medications that treat depression, Parkinson's disease, pain, and others. Not only does the type of neurochemical matter, but its location is also important for the resulting action. For example, opioids make one ignore pain and provide euphoria, but they also cause constipation acting on the receptors in the gut. In addition, the action of one neurochemical is almost always leads to modulation of other neurochemicals in this highly interconnected organ.

There are more than 60 chemicals identified as neurotransmitters. Sometimes, simple ions like zinc or nitric oxide as well as an electrical stimulus can be adequate for neurotransmission. The most common and relatively better-understood neurochemicals are amino acids such as glutamate or Gamma-Aminobutyric Acid (GABA), monoamines such as dopamine, adrenaline (epinephrine), serotonin, and histamine, and peptides like somatostatin, substance P, and endorphins.

Glutamate: Glutamate is the most abundant neurotransmitter in the brain. It is found in protein-rich foods and is believed to be responsible for the umami taste of meat. MSG or Mono-Sodium Glutamate, the food additive, is a levo isomer of glutamate. Glutamate is an excitatory neurotransmitter that seems to play a major role in learning and memory.

It is intracellular and is released during an injury, which can further harm the cell. Too much glutamate can cause seizures and death, and too little can also be harmful. Glutamate deficiency is associated with schizophrenia.

GABA: GABA is the inhibitory sibling of glutamate and is also abundant in the brain. It is generally associated with a calming effect, and so, a lack thereof is associated with anxiety and anxiety disorders. Calming drugs such as alcohol, barbiturates, and benzodiazepines act on GABA, and presumably, play a role in addiction. GABA is believed to play a role in brain development and maturation, and so, may be involved in a range of mental illnesses.

Dopamine: Well known for reduced levels resulting in Parkinson's disease, dopamine is a widely studied neurotransmitter. It is considered one of the pleasure chemicals directly tied to the reward mechanism in the brain. It is believed to play a role in motivation, learning, decision making, attention, and memory. Excess dopamine is associated with psychosis and schizophrenia. It is probably associated with other mental illnesses such as addiction and depression as well.

Serotonin: Frequently associated with mood, serotonin seems to be involved in contentment, confidence, self-esteem, appetite, sleep, and memory. Low serotonin is attributed to depression and suicide, and an increase of serotonin is related to recovery from depression.

Adrenaline: Adrenaline, or norepinephrine, is a hormone as well as a neurotransmitter. Popularly associated with thrill-seeking activities (like skydiving) and stress, it is a lifesaver in an allergic reaction (anaphylaxis) or cardiac arrest. As a hormone, it readies our body for the "fight or flight" response and plays a crucial role in anxiety disorders and PTSD.

Histamine: Histamine is the substance that causes allergic reactions. Although no clear relationship to mental illness has been proven, the antihistaminic effect of a lot of medications leads to sedation, which may be beneficial for sleep.

Endorphins: Endorphins are opioid analogs secreted in the body which act as natural pain killers. They also produce euphoria and calming effects, which, in turn, lead to opioid addiction.

Endocannabinoids: endocannabinoids are compounds similar to THC (Tetrahydrocannabinol), the active ingredient of cannabis, and are considered to have a role in memory, mood, appetite, and pain .

Oxytocin: Oxytocin has become very popular recently and is believed to be responsible for love, trust, and bonding. For example, oxytocin increases when a mother or father is with their baby.

It is important to note that as we understand more about neurotransmitters and their role in mental illness and psychiatric symptoms, it opens up opportunities to manipulate them for the benefit of symptom reduction and potential cures. The brain is a highly interconnected organ, and modulation in any part of it may have consequences elsewhere making it complex, challenging, and interesting to study.

Chapter 5

Psychosis and Schizophrenia

Schizophrenia is a chronic disabling mental illness that afflicts about 1% of the population. Considered as a neurodevelopmental disorder, it starts in young adults, usually with a psychotic episode. The psychosis improves with treatment, but rarely goes into complete remission and at least some form of the symptoms and disability remain for the rest of their lives. While schizophrenia is a major psychotic disorder, psychosis can appear in a variety of conditions. In this chapter, I will discuss psychosis (a symptom or a syndrome, not necessarily a disease on its own) first and then schizophrenia.

Psychosis

Psychosis is a strikingly morbid mental condition that is frightening, disabling, and disturbing for the individual and bystander alike. We do not understand what goes on inside a brain with psychosis, but it shakes the core concept of the self and impairs the reasoning and logical thinking that makes us who we are. In addition, psychosis impacts perception, emotion, cognition, and behavior, transforming a reasonable individual into a bizarre one who defies logic.

Psychosis is a symptom or a collection of symptoms including delusions, hallucinations, and disorganized thinking. Patients with psychosis can become agitated, restless, and lack focus and direction. They may not sleep well and can become too disorganized even to take care of themselves. They lose the capacity to understand and lack the awareness that their thoughts and emotions are not reality based. Psychosis can occur in a variety of illnesses and may result from a range of physiological and psychological causes. Schizophrenia is a disorder in which psychosis is enduring and lifelong and so it is rather easy to diagnose, but the psychosis that occurs in non-schizophrenic conditions can be a bit confusing.

The term psychosis itself is often loosely used leading to further confusion. When the patient's only symptom is a hallucination, it may not be referred as psychosis. For example, people who lose eyesight can have visual hallucinations, more or less like the "Phantom Limb" but it is not psychosis[1]. Although an isolated hallucination may be disabling and require treatment, it is not necessarily considered as psychosis.

Brief psychosis can be caused by stimulants like methamphetamine or methylphenidate, and by psychological conditions such as extreme stress, trauma, bereavement, or other psychiatric disorders such as depression, bipolar illness, or PTSD. Even sleep deprivation and caffeine intoxication may cause psychosis, albeit transiently. Many medical illnesses, including brain tumors, stroke, dementia, Parkinson's disease, and hormonal disorders can cause psychosis. Delirium (see chapter 13) resembles psychosis but there are distinct differences.

Delirium is a frequent medical complication that occurs in post-operative patients or in dementia. Delirium results from a disturbance in the homeostasis of the brain. This can happen for a variety of reasons including post-operative period, infection, electrolyte disturbance, and alcohol or drug withdrawal. Patients with delirium can have visual and auditory hallucinations, behave in a bizarre and confused manner and can become violent. But, the context of this, i.e. the sudden appearance of this behavior in medically compromised patients should make one consider delirium. In addition to being transient, these patients may not exhibit other characteristics of psychosis such as a thought disorder or a thematic, well-formed delusion. Patients with delirium are almost always confused and disoriented to time, place, or person (disorientation rarely happens in psychosis or any mental illness, and organic pathology should be suspected when disorientation is seen). Their attention is significantly impaired (a typical bedside test is to ask them to subtract 7s from 100 or 3s from 30, which they seldom complete).

Psychosis can occur with depression and mania. For example, a person with depression may have negative thoughts to start with. But when the depression gets severe, those thoughts can become delusional and they may start having hallucinations that reflect this sentiment. Similarly, positive or grandiose delusional beliefs (i.e., "I am a rock star") and hallucinations with positive messages can occur in mania, generally when it is severe. When psychotic symptoms and their contents are related to and reflect their mood, they are referred to as mood-congruent psychosis. However, patients with mania or depression can also

---

1 About 60-80% of amputees feel a sensation from the missing limb.

have psychosis or their content unrelated to their mood; this is called mood incongruent psychosis. Well, I did not promise this to be easy or straightforward.

Schizophrenia

Schizophrenia is a common disease that afflicts about 1% of the population. Schizophrenia runs in families, and the chance of developing the illness increases as one gets genetically closer to an affected individual. Among siblings and offspring of a patient, the risk is about 10%, or about 10 times higher than the general population. If both parents have schizophrenia, the odds for the child is almost 40% or more. If an identical twin - who is an identical genetic copy - has schizophrenia, the odds for the other twin is about 50%, which raises interesting issues. Although genetically identical, gene expression may vary between the twins for biological or environmental reasons.

It is estimated that about 80% of the illness is biological or determined at the time of birth. At this point, all evidence suggests that multiple genes are involved in schizophrenia, similar to other complex polygenetic illnesses, such as diabetes. Interestingly, a lot of personal psychological attributes like temperament, attitude, as well as other mental illnesses seem to follow similar genetic principles.

Although it appears small, the environmental contribution is a critical area for research because it may lead to interventions that may help in prevention as well as in treatment. The environmental factors include chemical insults in the womb, birth injuries such as a forceps injury during delivery, to drugs used in teen years, or stress in the developmental age. They may affect the brain directly, impede its development, or modify the genes leading to an abnormal developmental path towards schizophrenia. But, one thing is clear: child rearing has no impact on the development of schizophrenia. In the 70s, there was a baseless theory that mothers "caused" schizophrenia and these mothers were falsely known as "schizophrenogenic mother."

Men develop schizophrenia earlier (between ages 15-25) than women (25-35) and it is rare before age 15 or after age 50. Long before developing schizophrenia, children show subtle cognitive abnormalities such as poor fine motor coordination, language difficulties (especially receptive language abnormality or poor comprehension), and even mild abnormalities in thought. Immediately before developing the first episode of psychosis, patients go through a period of vague symptoms including social withdrawal, minimal hallucinations, delusions, and academic failure. This period can last for six months or longer and is called prodrome (not to be confused with schizophreniform, which requires overt psychosis).

In the past few decades, researchers and clinicians around the world became interested in prodrome as a window of opportunity for intervention and possibly prevention. Treatment of prodrome with antipsychotics or with psychosocial intervention may or may not prevent conversion to schizophrenia, but it is an excellent opportunity for early intervention, which may help in the long-term outcome.

Causes

The pathophysiology of schizophrenia is unknown and very little is known about the brain abnormalities. In fact, it was so frustrating for the scientists trying to find a clue about the illness, a neuropathologist in the 70s commented that "schizophrenia is the graveyard of neuropathologists." It is clear that Dopamine plays a role in psychosis. Increasing dopamine in the brain causes most of the psychotic symptoms, and most antipsychotics block dopamine. NMDA is also considered to play a major role in schizophrenia on its own or through dopamine. Again, as the brain is an interconnected, dynamic organ, and disturbance in one area, network, or neurochemical can influence other areas.

Recent MRI research has found, that patients with schizophrenia as a group have smaller total brain volume and volume reduction in several key areas such as frontal lobe, temporal lobe, superior temporal gyrus, hippocampus or amygdala. These are differences in the average brain volumes of patients compared to group of age and sex matched individuals with no schizophrenia. These abnormalities are not distinct enough to help diagnose a single patient. Microscopically, the neurons show fewer connections, which may be attributed to the volume reduction. Also, the developmental theory of schizophrenia supposes that poor or fewer connections are the result of impaired pruning or maturation of the brain.

Sometimes schizophrenia can be easily diagnosed, even by an untrained examiner, because of a few striking abnormalities including, disorganized or bizarre appearance or behavior, a significant reduction of emotional expression and social interaction, and a disconnectedness from their immediate surroundings. However, when asked to explain the core pathology in psychosis, even healthcare professionals have difficulty. It is helpful to think that psychosis is a disturbance in the thinking part or thought network of the brain, and schizophrenia is a disease of that network as opposed to depression or bipolar disorder, which involve the emotional part of the brain. But, as we discussed earlier, the brain is a highly interconnected organ and understandably, thought, emotion, and memory are connected and are dependent on each other. Even a loose definition of a specific network, region, or a connectome[2] to denote a complex brain function such as thought, or emotion may prove to be difficult.

When de novo psychosis occurs for less than a month, it is diagnosed as Brief Psychotic Disorder. The diagnostic criteria require delusions, hallucinations, disorganized speech and behavior. These patients generally do not have the chronic symptoms of schizophrenia like negative symptoms. A diagnosis of Schizophreniform disorder is offered for people who have psychosis for more than a month, but less than six months and the criteria include negative symptoms. Schizophreniform disorder is essentially a provisional diagnosis for schizophrenia, and if patients continue to have the symptoms beyond six months, they are diagnosed with schizophrenia.

Symptoms

A patient with schizophrenia experiences a variety of symptoms including hallucinations or false perceptions like hearing voices that are not there, delusions or false fixed beliefs, disorganized speech or behavior, and negative symptoms. The negative symptoms refer to something that is lost, like poor speech, inadequate emotional expression, and inactivity or lack of interest. They also suffer significant cognitive deficits that puts them at least a standard deviation below in IQ testing compared to their premorbid level. In addition to these symptoms, an important and common attribute of this illness is a lack of insight. People suffering from schizophrenia typically do not see their symptoms as abnormal and a result of a mental illness. Poor insight is one of the most common symptoms of schizophrenia, and a clinician would be very suspicious of the diagnosis if a patient has full insight. For some reason, the DSM committee does not seem to be impressed with lack of insight as a diagnostic criterion.

Some believe that schizophrenia is the severest illness to afflict mankind. I personally agree with this idea because this illness typically affects someone in the prime of their life and steals their thought, identity and feelings. Although it is not a deadly disease, it certainly takes the living out of life.

Hallucinations

Hallucinations are "false perceptions," meaning one perceives something without a stimulus. In schizophrenia, hearing voices is the

---

2 Connectome is a wordplay of genome and connections. It implies that a specific connection or network in the brain that may be responsible for a brain function and so an abnormality of the brain.

most common and well-known hallucination, but hallucinations can occur in all sensory modalities. Visual hallucinations are common or predominant in organic conditions such as delirium or seizures. Predominant olfactory hallucinations are frequently seen in temporal lobe epilepsy, but they can also occur in schizophrenia. Tactile hallucinations are feeling something on the skin (like bugs crawling). A hallucination can occur as a result of any disturbance in the neural pathway, like a tumor in the auditory nerve. In general, if the sensory end organs like the retina are affected, the patients see lights, sparks, or shadows, and if the cortex is affected, they see well formed, meaningful, complex figures and objects or people. Such isolated organic hallucinations without delusions or thought disorders are not usually identified as psychoses. Hallucinations could be a false perception of the patient's own thoughts, but it is not something they imagine, and it is not under their control. Quite often, a patient with schizophrenia, whose thought, and belief system are also affected, would believe, listen, and even follow the hallucinations, whereas someone who hears a sound caused by a tumor, would complain about the sound as abnormal and seek help. Sometimes non-psychotic patients may incorporate the organic voices into their belief system and may appear to be psychotic[3].

Delusion

A delusion is a fixed, false belief that is out of cultural norms. Delusions are common in schizophrenia, but they are neither essential nor sufficient for schizophrenia as they can often occur with other conditions such as depression or mania. Common delusional beliefs include conspiracy theories (people are plotting against me) or religious beliefs (I am sent by God for a purpose). "Ideas of reference" are false interpretations where the patient may believe that ordinary things have a special or exclusive meaning. For example, they may think that the doctors are wearing ties because they are listening to their thoughts.

A "Delusional Disorder" is an isolated delusion that does not (usually) occur with hallucinations or thought disorder. Patients affected by a delusional disorder are usually not as impaired in other functions and often maintain a successful personal and professional life. They may live with one odd belief all their lives and typically would refuse to seek help as the sole delusion may not cause significant impairment. Traditionally it is believed that these patients cannot be treated, but there is

[3] About 1 to 3 percent of people with temporal lobe epilepsy have religious experiences. It is believed that stimulation of the temporal lobe, especially on the right side makes one feel spiritual and feel, see or hear God. Some patients end up believing that they are God or God's messenger. Does this mean religion is "all in our head?" Maybe or maybe not. If we feel love for someone, it is mediated through neurotransmitters in the brain, but would it mean love is just in the head?

evidence that some patients improve with psychotherapy and medications.

Thought Disorder

The term schizophrenia was coined by Eugen Bleuler, who believed that the illness results from a split of the thinking mind and emotions. It has nothing to do with the popular mistaken reference of "split personality." Bleuler believed that abnormality of the thought is the core pathology in schizophrenia, which he explained results from impaired associations. A thought can be defined as a logical flow of ideas towards a specific goal. Bleuler explained that thought disoeder can result from poor or loose connections (associations) between the ideas. In addition to having disorganized thought, the patients may lack ideational richness, which is called poverty of content of thought. The patients are generally unaware of disorganized thinking and may at times, report jumbled up or racing thoughts. Please note that patients complain about "racing thoughts" in a variety of conditions including anxiety, mania and psychosis. Anxious patients are still organized in their thoughts and can redirect them. Manic patients jump from one topic to another known as "flight of ideas."

Negative Symptoms

As mentioned above, these are referred to as negative as they denote a lack or loss of function, as opposed to positive symptoms such as hallucinations and delusions, which would not happen normally. They include Alogia (poor speech), Affective flattening, avolition (lack of ability to plan or do useful activities), and anhedonia (lack of enjoyment).

Insight

A lack of insight or awareness of illness is highly prevalent in schizophrenia. Once again, this is an intriguing and interesting phenomenon that is hard to understand. The patients would have completely illogical thoughts and beliefs with no tangible evidence but cannot be convinced otherwise. They may not sleep for days and feel very scared but will refuse to get help. They would vehemently deny that they have a mental illness and deny that their thinking is in any way abnormal or illogical. It is similar to the neurological condition known as "anosognosia," which means a lack of knowledge or awareness.

Anosognosia is common in right-sided stroke involving fronto-parietal lobe. They are frequently unaware of their stroke and even when they acknowledge the stroke, they speak with an interesting indifference as if it does not belong to them, such as "Brian's leg doesn't work because of a stroke." It sometimes would appear that they possess the information but do not appreciate it.

While the degree of insight may vary in schizophrenia, a full and complete insight is rare and if they have full awareness of their symptoms it should prompt the clinician to look for organic causes such as brain pathology. Interestingly, improvement in insight is frequently seen in a clinical setting as a sign of improvement with treatment, but it is not frequently measured in clinical trials. Even when they gain some insight, they still have difficulty accepting the fact. But, at the same time they also seem to be aware of their predicament at some level despite the conviction. For example, a patient who claims to be the president may stay in a group home all his life, although sometimes he may claim the keys to the White House, which will take him to the hospital.

Catatonia

This is an interesting symptom, that illustrates the mind body interplay. Catatonia is characterized by stiffness and rigidity of skeletal muscles to a point, the patient may stay in an awkward position for hours or even days. Along with psychosis, agitation and other symptoms of psychosis, the patients exhibit stiff muscles, slow movements and rigidity (called as lead pipe rigidity because it feels like bending a soft metal when you examine these patients' movements).

Treatment

Treatment of schizophrenia involves an accurate diagnosis, antipsychotic medications, and psychosocial intervention, including rehabilitation. Antipsychotics are the mainstay of the treatment in acute episodes as well as chronic management. In an acute episode, hospitalization may be required because the patient may be too disorganized, may act upon his delusions or hallucinations compromising safety.

The choice of antipsychotics is almost entirely based upon the doctor's preference or bias. In general, second-generation antipsychotics are preferred due to fewer side effects. It is also helpful to consider the historical evidence for an effective medication. Usually in the acute setting, patients may need a larger dose of antipsychotic and some additional medication for sleep.

Sleep and psychosis have interesting two-way relationship. Patients do not sleep well in an acute psychotic episode. Poor sleep can cause or worsen psychosis and it is an early sign of relapse. Good sleep is a major aspect of recovery from psychosis.

The list of antipsychotics is discussed in detail in a later chapter. Haloperidol, fluphenazine, and chlorpromazine are older antipsychotics. Haloperidol is a potent dopamine blocker and is highly sedating, so it is frequently used in acute settings. Due to the high incidence of EPS (extrapyramidal side effects like tremors), they are not popular. Risperidone behaves more or less like haloperidol but is tolerated better. Olanzapine and Quetiapine are sedating. Aripiprazole and Ziprasidone are non-sedating and do not cause major weight gain. The choice is based on the side effects and personal preference. In the long term, weight gain is a major problem, so weight neutral drugs are preferable.

Once the patient improves, they sometimes become less tolerant of the medication and may show more side effects. Most of the patients need or only tolerate a smaller dose of the antipsychotic medication for maintenance and relapse prevention. Schizophrenia is a lifelong illness, and without treatment, patients typically relapse. The relapse may happen in two weeks or two years, but it invariably happens if they stop the medications. Patients may feel better immediately after they stop the medication because of a lack of side effects, which encourages them to stop or skip medications, but they would eventually worsen and relapse.

Within antipsychotics, there is no significant superiority of one medication over the other. Often, what works for a given patient is probably the best medicine for that patient, but it may be difficult to find the right one. Although it is not proven that the patients could become "tolerant" of a medication or "the medicine to lose its efficacy," patients can relapse even while taking medication and frequently need a different medicine. But there are many patients who stay on the same medication at the same dosage for long periods of time.

Besides antipsychotic medication, there is no convincing evidence in terms of a significant therapeutic benefit from any other medication or non-medication treatment. Similarly, there is no compelling evidence supporting a benefit from the use of multiple drugs (combination antipsychotics or others). However, in practice, polypharmacy is common for a variety of reasons. Psychotherapy, in terms of support, education, and rehabilitation also helps.

Schizophrenia is a relapsing and remitting illness. Early intervention and aggressive treatment in the early years help patients reduce relapses and improve long-term morbidity. Multiple relapses, especially in the early years, lead to a poor, protracted, and long recovery period and poor outcome. The patients, in general, do not agree with treatment because of a lack of insight. Family members do not fully understand the illness and implications of the patient's behavior. It is important that they get all the support and education they need. Unfortunately, it is common for patients to stop the medication and relapse.

The long-term course of schizophrenia varies depending upon the severity of the illness, its response to medication, patient's level of compliance, and the disability they sustain. Some patients take daily medications and can maintain a normal life with jobs and family while some end up institutionalized for life. In general, late onset, female sex, better insight, higher premorbid functioning, sobriety, good support system, and fewer negative symptoms indicate good prognosis. Some individuals with sporadic form of the illness tend to do better than those with family history. If heavy substance use precedes psychosis and they remain sober after the illness, they seem to do much better.

Schizoaffective disorder

Somewhat vague in its criteria, this diagnosis is offered when a patient has symptoms of schizophrenia and bipolar disorder. Even around the time Kraepelin differentiated schizophrenia and bipolar are two different illnesses, people noted that some patients present with symptoms of both. Simple way to understand this is to imagine a patient with both illnesses – enduring psychosis and acute psychotic, manic or depressive episodes. The key here is that the psychosis needs to be present for at least for two weeks or longer, independent of manic or depressive episodes. There are two subtypes, bipolar and depressive reflecting on the possibility of a bipolar illness or unipolar depression overlapping with schizophrenia. Due to the lack of clarity schizoaffective disorder is overdiagnosed. The treatment depends on the presence of mania or depression and they may need a mood stabilizer or antidepressant along with antipsychotics. The principles of managing a bipolar patient applies here. The disorder is much less common than diagnosed.

Five S's of Wellbeing[4]
1) Do not stop medication
2) do not use street drugs
3) sleep regularly,
4) use good support system and,
5) avoid or handle stress better.

---

[4] Thanks to Dr. Matcheri Keshavan, a great mentor, teacher and a master of acronyms.

Chapter 6

Mood Disorders

Mood is defined as the state of mind. Mood can be altered, at times very easily, by internal or external events, in a voluntary or involuntary manner. It can influence almost everything we do: our thinking, behavior, attitude, and productivity. The limbic system, a wide network of interconnected cortical and subcortical structures, is responsible for mood and its maintenance. This is a very complex system that connects almost every aspect of the brain function, from thought to bodily functions, like heart rate and breathing. The limbic system keeps our mood at an astonishingly stable level, varying with happiness and sadness within an acceptable range by the minute, by the day, by the year and over the lifetime. Without variations in mood, we would be like robots. Without feeling joy for happy times and despair during disappointments, our lives would have no motivation for success and no fear of failure, which would make life lifeless. The complexity of the limbic system and its connections can explain the role of mood and its impact on various mental illnesses. Mood disturbance is a component of many, if not all, mental illnesses, and mood disorders can influence or cause symptoms in thought and behavior.

Disorders of mood include: 1) depression, a persistent low mood for no apparent reason, 2) dysthymia, a long term, enduring, but a milder level of depression 3) bipolar disorder, characterized by episodes of depression and mania, and 4) cyclothymia, a weaker cousin of bipolar with milder highs and milder lows. The DSM-IV had depression and bipolar together as mood disorders but DSM-5 separated them, considering the possibility that bipolar illness may be distinct from other mood disorders. The DSM-5 also includes premenstrual dysphoric disorder in the depression section. For convenience and simplicity bipolar is included in this section.

Major Depressive Disorder (MDD)

Major depressive disorder is frequently referred to as "depression," "clinical depression," or "unipolar depression." When I say depression in this context, I refer to a distinct disease (or a disorder) of mood, in which one has persistent, pervasive low and sad mood associated with other symptoms as explained in the diagnostic criteria. It also implies that depression needs intervention, would respond to medication, and, if left untreated, it might worsen to a point where the patients may endanger their lives with neglect and/or suicide.

However, quite often, the distinction between depression as a disease and someone's bad or sad mood may not be clear. In the past, some believed that there was this "endogenous depression" which is more of a brain disorder as opposed to a "reactive depression" that could be an individual's reaction to some unfortunate circumstances. While there may be some truth to this distinction, such thinking can be confusing and misleading, especially in the choice of treatment. Sometimes patients, their relatives, as well as professionals may erroneously believe that such a "reactive" depression is under the individual's control and, therefore, they expect them just to shake it off - leading to under-diagnosis and under-treatment.

Until there is a clear lab test that helps us diagnose depression as a disease, it is better to err on the safe side of treating the depression even when the presentation is not very convincing. Everyone with a persistent sad mood needs help. This could be emotional support for a friend in tough times, psychotherapy, or medications, depending upon the situation. Considering the cost-benefit ratio, there is very little to lose with any of these simple interventions, including medications, which are generally or relatively harmless. In addition, considering the subjective nature of the symptoms and the unclear boundary between normal and abnormal, it is not a bad idea to have an open mind while dealing with depression and offer help to a suffering and help-seeking patient, as long as there is no harm done.

Because of this, one can presume that depression may be over-diagnosed at least in some settings. However, this is one of the most under-diagnosed illnesses for a variety of reasons. It is estimated that about 50 to 70% of the patients with depression are not recognized in the primary care setting. This could be due to the patient's lack of awareness, understatement of the symptoms, denial, or stigma. Even when they indicate their emotional problems, the busy clinicians are often reluctant to discuss emotional issues. The clinician may feel uncomfortable, lack adequate training or experience, or not have enough time. But things are changing with better training for the primary care physicians and with the introduction of SSRIs, which are a lot easier to prescribe and monitor than older medications. Nowadays, a lot of patients are diagnosed and appropriately treated in the primary care setting. Yet, it is true that even when recognized, some patients refuse to take the medications, and even after they are prescribed, they may not fill them or take them long enough to get an adequate response. Depression is an easily diagnosable and treatable disease, but it still remains as one of the most burdensome illnesses for the society according to WHO.

A depressive episode is a distinctive period of sadness that is unmistakable as a clinically abnormal state of mind at its peak, but it may creep in slowly without the awareness of the patient or family. What appears to be a bad day might turn out to be a bad week, then a bad month, and so on. The patients may readily acknowledge the deep suffering and the psychological pain of depression, but they often incorporate the disease state into their sense of self, at times denying the illness and blaming themselves. The diagnostic criteria need an episode of distinct and abnormal sadness that lasts for at least two weeks or more in which five of the following nine symptoms occur: depressed or sad mood most of the day, a significant lack of interest in activities, unintended weight loss or gain, insomnia or hypersomnia, psychomotor retardation or agitation, fatigue or loss of energy, feelings of worthlessness, helplessness or hopelessness, poor concentration, and thoughts of death or suicide.

Some patients tend to report more physical symptoms such as fatigue, low energy, and aches and pains. This is seen more frequently among women, children, and the elderly, but men who do not want to admit or accept a sad mood may also report physical symptoms. Perception, self-assessment, and linguistic sophistication may affect the reporting of the symptoms which need to be considered in the evaluation of a patient. Some patients may report anxiety as the major presenting symptom.

While assessing or understanding the person with depression, it is important to remember that these symptoms, alone or together, can occur in a number of situations that may not constitute clinical depression. For example, grief and severe losses in life such as losing a job or one's life savings can lead to a state of sadness. When the depression occurs in the presence of a significant life event, symptoms need to be disproportionately severe or longer. In other words, if the depression is severe enough, it should be treated appropriately despite the circumstances. Depression is often precipitated by life events and, not infrequently, the patients with depression get themselves into major life crises because of the illness. For example, an individual with depression could lose their job due to poor performance, which compounds the problem.

Like most of the mental illnesses, genes play a major role in the susceptibility for MDD, but stressful life events, losses in life, and poor social support all seem to contribute to the occurrence of depression. In addition, physical illness and other mental illnesses including drug abuse and alcohol use increase the odds of developing depression. Around 10% of men and 20% of women seem to get MDD at least once in their lifetime. Depression is a critical healthcare problem in the general medical setting because it significantly interferes with medical illnesses. Having depression after a myocardial infarct increases the morbidity and doubles the death rate after having a heart attack. By the way, depression as a risk factor for coronary artery disease is as bad as high cholesterol.

The patients typically acknowledge their deep suffering and psychic pain readily but like many things in life, they tend to incorporate the disease state into themselves. Psychologically, the depression zaps the energy out of the patient's life and makes them see everything with a negative outlook - of themselves, their lives and their future. The negative outlook extends to an attitude of low self-worth, low self-confidence, poor and negative assessment of themselves, and their accomplishments. They develop a negative and adversarial outlook on their current surroundings as well as a pessimistic and hopeless attitude towards their future. An understanding of this cognitive process would help in treating a patient experiencing depression. Quite often, one can challenge these attitudes with facts, which almost always helps with a change of perspective. For example, someone with depression would frequently say that "my life is the worst and I am a total failure," but the wrong belief can often be challenged with facts, albeit very slowly. Such an approach used in a psychological treatment called CBT, or cognitive behavioral therapy.

Depression and chronic pain

There are evidence that chronic pain can lead to depression and chronic depression can cause or exacerbate pain. Pain has a major emotional component and, somehow, in the interconnected brain, depression and chronic pain reinforce each other.

Dysthymia

Dysthymia is a milder form of depression and is generally believed to be enduring, although it can ebb and flow. Dysthymia does not get as severe as the major depressive disorder, but the two can co-occur. Dysthymia was renamed as Persistent Depressive Disorder. For a diagnosis, the depressed mood is supposed to last for at least 2 years with at least two of the following symptoms: Poor appetite or overeating, insomnia or hypersomnia, low energy or fatigue, low self-esteem, poor concentration or difficulty making decisions, and feelings of hopelessness. The patients quite often consider these symptoms as part of themselves and may not complain about the chronic feeling of sad mood. The diagnostic criteria require no symptom-free period of 2 months or more, and for children, the duration requirement is 1 year. But, the essential feature of dysthymia that differentiates it from MDD is that this is milder but enduring. Children may report anger, pain, and irritability as the main features.

Depression in other illnesses

MDD can co-occur with almost any mental illness (schizophrenia, anxiety disorders, substance use, etc.). Personality disorders are frequently encountered in the clinical setting with a complaint or a diagnosis of MDD. These patients, including patients with borderline personality disorder, report a chronic and enduring but not episodic feeling of emptiness with mood swings or poor mood regulation. The treatment is the same as MDD along with addressing the co-morbid illness.

Postpartum Depression

There is an increased vulnerability for women to develop depression, mania, psychosis, and other mental illnesses after childbirth. Quite often, childbirth seems to precipitate first episode of these illnesses in some women. Twenty percent or one in five new mothers experience some form of psychological symptoms that may need treatment. These could be new episodes, one-time episodes, or relapse of a chronic illness. Sometimes, a severe form of the postpartum depression may start during pregnancy. Postpartum depression is treated in the same way as depression.

Premenstrual Dysphoric Disorder (PMDD)

PMDD is not the same as premenstrual syndrome or PMS. PMS is a milder form. PMDD is sometimes referred to as "Late Luteal-phase Dysphoric Disorder." A typical menstrual cycle starts after the menses with the secretion of estradiol, which primes the uterus, and at about mid-cycle, an increase in estradiol leads to a surge of Luteinizing hormone (LH surge) which results in ovulation and release of the egg from the ovarian follicle. The remnants of the follicle become a structure called the corpus luteum that secretes progesterone, which prepares the endometrium for the reception of zygote in the uterus if the egg is fertilized. If the egg does not get fertilized, the corpus luteum slowly reduces the amount of progesterone it secretes, and the cycle ends in the next month's menses. It is this period, at about 4 to 7 days before the menses, when PMS and PMDD occur as if the uterus is disappointed that fertilization did not occur.

The DSM criteria for PMDD is a bit confusing. However, the timing of these symptoms, starting within a week before the onset of menses that stop or reduce significantly at the onset or immediately after the onset of menses should alert the clinician. It requires presence of five or more of the following symptoms: affective lability/mood swings, irritability/anger, depressed mood, or anxiety/tension, decreased interest in day to day things, difficulty with concentration, lack of energy or fatigue, change in appetite, sleep problems, sense of being overwhelmed or out of control, and physical symptoms such as breast tenderness, joint pain, bloated feeling or weight gain.

PMDD occurs in about 5% of women. Sometimes, this can be disabling. It is also estimated that up to 80% of women experience some symptoms of irritability or tension building up before the periods. The PMS, a lighter version of PMDD, occurs in about one in four to one in three women. SSRIs are used during the premenstrual time with some success. Benzodiazepines also have a good response. Some patients with generalized anxiety disorder or major depressive disorder cycle through the month with worsening symptoms during the premenstrual time.

Treatment of MDD

The mainstay of treatment of MDD is antidepressants. A number of psychotherapy techniques work very well and among them, CBT, or cognitive behavioral therapy, is a bit more structured and predictable. The effectiveness of St. John's wort in depression is debatable, but it seems that it helps milder depression (not necessarily dysthymia), but not moderate or severe forms of depression.

Among antidepressants, the selective serotonin reuptake inhibitors (SSRIs) are the most popular. These are convenient, taken once a day, have minimal need for dose adjustment (several of them work at 20 mg), and are generally tolerated well. Popular SSRIs include fluoxetine, paroxetine, citalopram, escitalopram (all therapeutic dose of about 20 mg) and sertraline (50 mg). SSRIs increase inter-cellular serotonin by reducing the reuptake, which is one of the ways the neurons modulate the level of neurochemicals in the synapse. It is commonly believed that an increase in serotonin results in an improvement of depression, although it is unclear how these medications work. Serotonin is an interesting neurochemical that is also present abundantly in the gut and controls gut motility. Low serotonin is associated with low confidence, suicide, obsessive compulsive disorder, and even falling in love. I am not making any assumptions here about depression and falling in love, but it is believed that the anxiety and obsessive behavior around falling in love is related to the lowering of serotonin level.

Tricyclic antidepressants such as imipramine, amitriptyline, nortriptyline, trimipramine, and doxepin are older medications that have more side effects and need complex dose adjustments. SNRIs (serotonin and norepinephrine reuptake inhibitors) are another group of medications that increase or modulate both serotonin and norepinephrine and thus provide antidepressant effect (at some point, norepinephrine was considered as the key neurotransmitter involved in depression). SNRIs include duloxetine and venlafaxine. Desvenlafaxine, another SNRI, is the active metabolite of venlafaxine. Many practitioners use SNRIs as the second line medication when SSRIs fail. The SNRIs also help in chronic pain and are preferred when pain and depression occur together. Bupropion works through dopamine and has a mild stimulant effect. Because of this, it is frequently used for patients who complain of low energy, motivation, and concentration. It also helps in quitting smoking.

MAOIs (monoamine oxidase inhibitors) are somewhat complex medications that cause severe side effects, and so are reserved as the last resort medications for the treatment of depression. These drugs (selegiline, moclobemide, rasagiline, isocarboxazid, phenelzine, tranylcypromine) are excellent antidepressants. Monoamine oxidase is an enzyme that breaks down monoamines and by blocking the enzyme, these drugs increase the availability of monoamines such as serotonin or norepinephrine. The notable side effect of these medications is a hypertensive crisis resulting from the ingestion of foods rich in tyramine such as cheese or fermented foods (cheese effect). Tyramine is normally broken down at the liver by MAO and MAOIs block MAO, leading to accumulation of high levels of tyramine in the blood. Tyramine is believed to replace and release excessive norepinephrine, which causes a hypertensive crisis. This reaction is variable and unpredictable but can be life-threatening, which scares patients and doctors alike. MAOIs are believed to help people with atypical depression as well as panic disorder, anxiety disorders, OCD, and bulimia.

Augmentation of Antidepressants

A substantial portion of patients do not get better with the first trial of antidepressants. They need to switch to a different class or add another treatment, especially for those who respond partially. Sometimes an increase in the dose works but many may require augmentation. Such augmentation strategy could be addition of another medication such as buspirone, bupropion, or psychotherapy such as Cognitive Behavioral Therapy (CBT). Lithium carbonate at a smaller dose of 300 mg (compared to the typical mood stabilizer dose of 900 mg or so, decided by the blood level) or triiodothyronine (T3, a thyroid supplement) are frequently used in addition to antidepressants. These two are proven to make the antidepressants work better, particularly among partial responders.

Using antipsychotics as augmentation agents for depression has become popular these days. Personally, I have some hesitation in using antipsychotics in non-psychotic patients due to the side effects. If a patient with depression happens to have psychosis, antipsychotics can and probably should be used along with the antidepressants, at least until the psychosis clears. But, for depression, it is much better to try all other medication options before trying antipsychotics. Antipsychotics have severe side effects compared to SSRIs, and the evidence in the literature is mostly on the depression that occurs in bipolar disorder rather than unipolar depression. Patients with MDD who take antipsychotics are susceptible for tardive dyskinesia (a movement disorder).

Ketamine, an anesthetic has been found to help patients with MDD. Recently S-ketamine, an isomer of Ketamine, is approved by the FDA for treatment-resistant depression. Ketamine is an NMDA antagonist and it seems to help improve mood within a day or so. This is a revolutionary new treatment. As a controlled substance, its use is restricted and needs to follow strict guidelines. Trans cranial magnetic stimulation and vagal nerve stimulation are newer treatment modalities that are proven to help depression.

Electro-convulsive Therapy (ECT)

ECT is one of the oldest treatments in mental health. In 1930s, Ladislas Meduna, a Hungarian psychiatrist believed that seizures and schizophrenia operate opposite to each other because he noticed schizophrenia patients getting better after they have seizures from an unrelated reason[1]. He induced seizures by injecting camphor and found patients with catatonia improve. Ugo Cerletti and Lucio Bini in Italy introduced electricity to induce seizures. Although it was used in psychosis earlier, ECT is an excellent treatment for severe depression and catatonia. In a typical ECT treatment, electrical stimulus is applied at the temple bilaterally or unilaterally to induce the seizure under general anesthesia. It is given in a course of 6 to 12 treatments or until the patient improves. Some patients benefit from weekly maintenance ECTs. ECT is safe and complications generally arise from the anesthesia. Cognitive deficits

---

1 Patients with epilepsy, sometimes develop psychosis in late 20s and they were noted to improve in their psychosis after having a seizure.

and confusion can occur immediately after treatment, but they get better over time.

STAR*D trial is a famous large study of treatment of depression in the primary care setting. About 4000 patients were enrolled, and about 2800 patients were treated and observed. Initially (level 1), they were given citalopram, an SSRI, and, after about six weeks, a third had remission and became symptom-free. In addition, about 10-15% had good improvement. Those who did not improve were offered either a switch to a different medication (sertraline, bupropion-SR or venlafaxine-XR) or added another medication (bupropion or buspirone) or given a choice to add CBT or switch to CBT. In level 2, another 25% attained remission. People who had severe side effects opted to switch as opposed to add on. In level 3, those who did not respond in level 2 were given the option to add either lithium or thyroxine or switch to different drugs (mirtazapine or nortriptyline). A further 12 to 20% improved with no significant difference between the options. People who took lithium experienced more side effects than the thyroid hormone. Those who did not respond were assigned to level 4, in which they were given either an MAOI or a combination of mirtazapine and venlafaxine, which helped another 10%.

The study implies that some medications are better than others. However, this is a naturalistic "study," which is informative to the extent that the design is the result. The design reflects the belief and recommendation of the experts partly based on the side effects or risk-benefit ratio and includes all scientific evidence and well-educated guesses. It is quite possible that some patients respond to certain medication better than others, so it is disputable to claim that one medication is better than the other. What works best for one person is not necessarily the best for others. The trick is to find the one that works for each person. This is a major area of clinical and scientific interest. Choice of drugs can be based on past history of response, family history, symptomatology (atypical symptoms such as hypersomnia respond well to unusual drugs like bupropion), safety profile, patient preference, pharmacogenetics, and more. (See the section of psychopharmacology for more information about medication.)

Bipolar Disorder

Bipolar disorder is a fascinating illness. Characterized by episodes of depression and mania, it can cause significant suffering, loss, and long term disability. But, unlike schizophrenia, many patients with bipolar are relatively higher functioning and can lead a reasonably normal life, at least in between episodes. In fact, many individuals with bipolar lead more productive lives than the rest of us. People with bipolar do not always fit the stereotype of the mentally ill, who are often perceived or portrayed as dysfunctional, fearsome, disconnected, and unlikeable individuals. Instead, patients with bipolar are quite often charming, pleasant, and are a joy to be with, especially when they are manic or hypomanic. Mania is often referred to as a high without drugs. While manic, patients may enjoy every minute of their mania but bipolar disorder is not fun to have.

At the outset, it may appear to be simple and easy to conceptualize or understand mood disorders, meaning one is abnormally, excessively, and pathologically sad in depression and abnormally, excessively, and pathologically happy in mania, and when they cycle through these abnormal ups and downs (in their lifetime), we know they have bipolar disorder. However, quite often, the patients show up with a complex presentation, history, and course of illness that makes it difficult to understand and diagnose. In addition, a patient's other comorbid problems such as drug and alcohol use, life stressors, and additional symptoms such as anxiety or side effects of medications can add to the confusion. A lack of clear understanding of mood episodes, a lack of clear boundary between normal and abnormal highs and lows, as well as symptomatic overlap with other illnesses like schizophrenia confuse further.

It is very important to understand the difference between the day-to-day variation of mood or mood instability and the real mania and depression. Say, for example, we normally have a certain degree of ups and downs in our mood over any given period of time - within a day or a year or in our lifetime. Some of us may have a bit higher ups and lower lows and some may have better control or regulation of the ups and downs. These variations between individuals are generally determined by personality, age, social, and cultural settings, and quite often these may, at most, cause minor inconveniences in life but not lead to a full-blown disability.

In contrast, the bipolar disorder causes the individual to go through a state of "super happiness" for a sustained period of time, typically weeks and months and similar periods of extreme sadness that are pathological and clearly beyond normal experiences. In addition, these manic and depressive "states of mind" typically last for a few weeks to few months each - not (usually) hours or days. Bipolar disorder is frequently confused with borderline personality disorder in which mood change is apparent within minutes or hours, usually due to an identifiable internal or external reason. It is also common for laypeople to refer to their mood changes - usually anger - as having bipolar. It is important to understand the symptoms to make a clear diagnosis, at least in the classic patients. There are always exceptions and variabilities, which I will discuss later.

Mania

A manic episode is defined by a distinct period of persistently elevated mood that lasts for at least one week according to the DSM-5 criteria. The criteria also require three of the following: inflated self-esteem, decreased need for sleep, pressured speech, flight of ideas, distractibility, increased goal-directed activity, and poor judgment leading to indulgence in activities that might cause harm later.

The key here is an abnormal or pathological and persistent elevation of mood. Even extreme happiness that one might enjoy on occasions (for tangible reasons) might pale in comparison to the manic state of mind these patients experience. They call it a high without drugs for a reason. The criteria have a 7-day requirement for the diagnosis of mania, but they can last for a few days to few months or longer, with some patients experiencing occasional, unexplainable bouts of happiness for a few days. A manic individual may be charming, gregarious, seductive, creative, full of tireless energy needing only two or three hours of sleep and may start multiple projects with great ideas, and sometimes be successful. But almost always at some point, the mania impairs the judgment of the person and they end up doing things that they would not otherwise do, such as shopping sprees or sexual indiscretions. Often the patients who go through mania do not realize it is abnormal and take on the ride readily. Unlike the lack of insight in schizophrenia, patients who are manic may (sometimes)acknowledge that they are not normal but might resist the idea that it is a disorder. They are like a hurricane with matching judgment and insight.

Mania and hypomania are treated with mood stabilizers (lithium, valproate, carbamazepine, oxcarbazepine, or lamotrigine) and/or antipsychotics. In acute settings sedating antipsychotics such as olanzapine, quetiapine or haloperidol are preferred.

Bipolar depression

A bipolar depressive episode is similar to the MDD discussed earlier. The diagnostic criteria need an episode of distinct and abnormal sadness that lasts at least two weeks or more in which five of the following nine symptoms are present: Depressed or sad mood most of the day, a significant lack of interest in activities, unintended weight loss or gain, insomnia or hypersomnia, psychomotor retardation or agitation, fatigue or loss of energy, feelings of worthlessness, helplessness or hopelessness, poor concentration, and thoughts of death or suicide.

Clinically, an episode of bipolar depression may be indistinguishable from a unipolar depression and they are treated in the same way. It is important to keep in mind that they can become manic or hypomanic as they improve with treatment. So, one needs to obtain the past history and family history for mania, especially at the first time. They should remain or be started on a mood stabilizer. If the patient has a history of treatment and benefit from an antipsychotic, it may help preventing mania as well as helping with depression.

The bipolar depression starts at a younger age, may have shorter episodes, that worsen or improve in a faster pace compared to unipolar depression. They also have fewer anxiety symptoms. Family history is important to consider when treating depression. However, it is also true that unipolar depression is more common in family members of patients with bipolar illness. Who said psychiatry was easy?

Hypomania

Hypomania is a less intense form of mania. The DSM criteria require a persistent and abnormal elevated mood or irritability and increased activity or energy that lasts at least 4 consecutive days. They are also required to have three of the following symptoms: inflated self esteem, decreased need for sleep, being talkative, flight of ideas, distractibility, increase in goal directed activity and engaging in activities that may lead to negative consequences. These symptoms must be observable as more than their normal asymptomatic state. If these symptoms are severe enough to the point of marked disability to the point of hospitalization or presence of psychosis the episode must be diagnosed as mania. A patient who has only hypomanic episode will be diagnosed with bipolar II. Patients with bipolar I can also have hypomanic episodes.

Rapid cycling and mixed episodes

If the patient has 4 identifiable episodes of mania, depression or hypomania, it is known as rapid cycling. If a manic patient, has some symptoms of depression, it is identified as mixed episode. The day to day mood changes of personality disorder is often mis-identified as rapid cycling.

Diagnostic Challenges in Bipolar Illness

Bipolar disorder is one of the most over-diagnosed illnesses in clinical practice. This is due to mis-identification of short term well being or irritability as hypomania. Overlapping mood changes of personality disorder is also misdiagnosed as rapid cycling bipolar.

Mood Disorders

Psychosis and bipolar

This is a bit complex. In simple terms, a patient in a depressive episode or a manic episode can have psychotic symptoms, particularly when the depression or mania is severe. Negative (or positive) thoughts of depression (or mania) can become more intense and become delusional. They can have hallucinations related to their mood or thought. These are known as mood congruent psychoses. They can also have psychosis that is not congruent (thematically unrelated) with the mood. Presence of psychosis generally implies the episode is severe. It appears that some bipolar patients are more susceptible to get psychotic symptoms than others. Some patients never experience psychosis and some present with psychosis independent of mood symptoms. When the psychosis happens independent of mood symptoms, they will be diagnosed with schizoaffective disorder.

One can imagine the variabilities you could see from a clean bipolar to a clean schizophrenia (if there are any of those) and a confusing mixture in between. It seems bipolar illness is more related to schizophrenia than unipolar depression but the issue is unsettled.

Treatment

An acute episode of depression in bipolar is treated like unipolar depression (with caution as mentioned above) and mania is treated with antipsychotics and mood stabilizers. Long term maintenance of these patients generally require close monitoring.

Although the treatment of bipolar disorder may seem straightforward, and some patients do live well with just one mood stabilizer such as lithium for long periods of time, bipolar is frequently a challenge in the outpatient setting. This could be due to complexities in the presentation, treatment response, and comorbidities. In general, a patient with bipolar disorder should be on a mood stabilizer such as lithium, valproic acid (Depakote), carbamazepine, oxcarbazepine, or lamotrigine. A manic patient would need an antipsychotic along with a mood stabilizer, and they should not be taking an antidepressant when flagrantly manic. When a patient is depressed, they need an antidepressant, but it is prudent to keep them on a mood stabilizer and watch them closely for mania. (See psychopharmacology chapter for more details).

The most important thing in the management of bipolar besides the medication is sleep. Lack of sleep can precipitate mania and quite often poor sleep is an early indicator of forthcoming mania. Substance abuse and stress can also precipitate manic or depressive episodes.

Patients need education, support and psychotherapy to handle the stress associated with the illness and management of symptoms.

Confusing Things About Bipolar Disorder

1. Normal or extreme normal mood swings are not bipolar.
2. Mood instability or poor control of mood is not necessarily bipolar.
3. One manic episode should be diagnosed with bipolar.
4. Multiple depressive episodes with no manic episode should be characterized as unipolar depression until they develop mania. A family history of bipolar should be a caution flag.
5. In general, an abnormal "happiness" is required to have mania. But there are exceptions.
6. True rapid cycling and mixed episodes are rare - and mood swings of personality disorders are frequently mistaken by the patients as well as clinicians as these.
7. It is very common for patients and clinicians to misdiagnose personality disorders as bipolar disorder.
8. There is so much overlap between bipolar and other illnesses, including personality disorders, schizophrenia, and anxiety disorder that even a seasoned clinician can make mistakes.
9. There seems to be a biological, genetic, and symptomatic overlap of several diagnoses.
10. The treatment also causes confusion:
- Bipolar with depression can become manic (including for the first time) with antidepressant treatment.
- Lithium is a good mood stabilizer for bipolar, it is a good anti manic, and it works well as an augmentation agent for depression.
- Most of the antipsychotics work as antimanics
- Some of the newer antipsychotics work for bipolar depression (and are frequently used in unipolar depression with or without evidence).
- Many patients end up with one medication from each class - and as unintelligent as it seems, this strategy seems to work for many patients.
- However, it is very important NOT to give antidepressants to patients in mania.

Chapter 7

Anxiety Disorders

Anxiety is uncomfortable even when it is about something nice, say, for example, waiting for your first date. But why do we have to feel uncomfortable when anticipating something pleasant and exciting? We feel anxious and apprehensive when the outcome is important but uncertain, whether it is pleasant or unpleasant. Such anxiety helps us by increasing focus to do our best on the task at hand to achieve the best outcome and avoid the worst. We try our best to make sure the date goes well so that we don't miss out on the opportunity to court the man or woman of our dreams (or avoid a disaster that may haunt the rest of our lives). Fear is somewhat distinct from anxiety in that it is a response to an impending threat, either real or perceived. Fear and anxiety are self-preserving and essential for our survival, whether it is in a cave in the jungle or in a suburban home with a CCTV. Evolution, through natural selection, preserved those characteristics that prolong and sustain life, whether it is the resilience of the bamboo in a windy region or the fear of predators in a desert.

Moderate anxiety is productive. There is an inverted U-shaped relationship between anxiety and performance. This connection is explained by two psychologists, Robert Yerkes and William Dodson, in 1908 as the Yerkes-Dodson law[1]. Arousal and anxiety at a moderate level improve performance. Anyone who played sports would know that the anxiety of the situation (popularly referred to as adrenaline rush) would propel them to do things they may not do otherwise. One needs at least some minimal fear of failure or embarrassment to motivate himself to perform well, but, if it becomes excessive, it could be crippling.

---

[1] Robert Yerkes was a Harvard professor who was famous for intelligence testing and primate behavior. The primate 'language' is named after him as Yerkish. Interestingly, he supported eugenics as his research "showed" immigrants to be less intelligent.

An uncomfortable but reasonably healthy level of anxiety, generally reflective of the danger one faces can manifest in day-to-day occasions such as exams, job interviews, or meeting that boy for the first time. Such situational anxiety is necessary, although it can be counterproductive at times. However, an anxiety disorder is a condition where the anxiety is completely unnecessary and often impedes and impairs the person's functioning, at times, to the point of total disability. Similar to how every system in the body built for a productive purpose can go wrong, when this system in the brain is disrupted, it can lead to several disorders. In this section, I will discuss generalized anxiety disorder, panic disorder, agoraphobia, social anxiety disorder, and OCD.

Generalized Anxiety Disorder

As the name implies, in this condition, the sufferer experiences excessive anxiety and worry about anything and everything in life. The patients often describe an inability to relax and feeling wound up with an exhausting and restless mind. These patients live like they are under severe stress all the time, while their life may not be any different from others. Even in the presence of stress, the worry or anxiety is out of proportion.

According to the DSM-5 diagnostic criteria, for a diagnosis of GAD, a patient should experience excessive anxiety and worry about multiple things in life for at least six months, occurring more than 50% of the days. They should have three of these six symptoms: restlessness (keyed up or on edge feeling), easy fatigue, difficulty in concentration, irritability, muscle tension, and poor sleep.

As in other conditions, an impairment (in social, personal, or professional life) is necessary for a diagnosis, and anxiety experienced in the context of another psychiatric or medical illness or drug use are excluded. Anxiety caused by other physical conditions such as drug use, drug withdrawal, or hormonal imbalance (hyperthyroidism and adrenal tumors that produce excessive corticosteroids) usually, but not always, subside when the primary cause is treated. There is a large component of "learning" in anxiety, and individuals who experience repeated stressful events can become conditioned to respond with excessive anxiety, even for day-to-day events.

The classic patient with GAD is easily recognizable and diagnosable, and they are also easy to treat in that they respond very well for antidepressants and CBT. A selective serotonin reuptake inhibitor like fluoxetine (Prozac), paroxetine, or citalopram works very well.

However, it is important to understand that anxiety as a symptom (as opposed to a disease of its own) can frequently occur in other conditions such as depression and OCD. Depression and anxiety go hand in hand. A lot of patients with depression have anxiety as a symptom, and patients with anxiety disorders report feeling depressed. Patients can have anxiety and depression together as two illnesses, two sides of the same illness, or symptoms of one another. For example, a patient with major depressive disorder can have anxiety as a dominant symptom along with sad mood, and a patient with GAD may walk into your office claiming that they are depressed. The constant worry of GAD sometimes may appear similar to depression and patients may even perceive it as depression. Diagnostically, it might confuse even the best in the field, but one can come to a fairly clear and confident conclusion by listening to the patient patiently to understand them. The longitudinal history and the qualitative and quantitative assessment of symptoms should help reach a clear diagnosis.

Personally, I emphasize giving a clear diagnosis, but more so, I think it is important to understand the symptoms and the psychology behind them. It is very important to have a clear idea of the patient and his or her perspective of their experiences. It is our job to explain and reassure patients about their symptoms and diagnosis. Whether the patient suffers from depression, anxiety, or OCD, the treatment is the same, i.e., they all can be helped by SSRIs, and therapy can focus on the specific symptom that is bothering the patient irrespective of the diagnosis.

CBT plays a significant role in symptom improvement in GAD. Relaxation techniques such as deep muscle relaxation, deep breathing, and exposure (to anxiety provoking situations) help improve symptoms. Propranolol or beta-blockers give good symptom relief without sedation or dependence. Twenty mg of propranolol once or twice a day as needed works well for most patients, especially around the time they are start taking an antidepressant.

Panic Disorder

A panic attack is anxiety unplugged. GAD is a constant, low-grade uncomfortable fear, or rather a nagging worry, but a panic attack is a full force torrent of fear that hits you from nowhere without a warning and for no reason. Quite often, people think that they are having a heart attack and end up in the hospital or they fear that they are going crazy. They usually remember every bit of the first attack of panic vividly for the rest of their lives.

The anxiety in a panic attack is explained as a "fear of impending doom." The unbearable fear and anxiety escalate with a multitude of physical symptoms, including palpitations or pounding in the heart, shortness of breath almost like an asthma attack, and feeling like they are being choked or smothered in addition to the feeling of being trapped. They hyperventilate, feel numbness and tingling sensations in their fingertips and experience paresthesias. They may shake in fear, feel dizzy, or lightheaded, but they do not typically lose consciousness, although it can happen. They describe butterflies in the stomach or a knot in the stomach that gets tighter by the minute and may feel nauseous. They feel hot and sweat profusely. Some patients describe the feeling as they have an intense desire to jump out of their imploding and painful bodies that are hot, trembling, and covered with sweat, but are unable to do so. Interestingly, some do feel depersonalization or an out-of-body experience that might not be a relief because they watch themselves breaking down and genuinely fear dying or losing their sanity.

As they go through a panic attack, and as the symptoms become unbearable, they may even think of death as a relief. The attack usually subsides in a few minutes, leaving the individual drained and exhausted. However, they are rather scarred for life from the dreadful experience. Even when it is over and even after the patient is reassured that there is nothing life-threatening, the panic attack leaves an indelible mark on their psyche. They remember and fear the panic attack itself. They start living with constant fearful anticipation of another attack. Now, they learn to fear the fear. Even if the attack happens rarely, they live in constant fear of getting another attack, and this fear changes their behavior, often drastically.

They stay home and refuse to venture into anything. Some may even dread getting out of the bedroom and coming to the living room to meet the rest of the family. They start living in constant fear of being ambushed by another panic attack. While knowing that this is a panic attack and not a heart attack gives them relief, they are now worried about the embarrassment of having a mini psychological breakdown in the presence of others. A panic attack is more embarrassing than a stroke because we humans are a lot more kind when the affliction is physical rather than psychological.

An attack of anxiety or a sudden increase in anxiety symptoms that is not a panic attack can happen to even otherwise stable individuals or among those suffering from other mental illnesses. Individuals with depression or GAD are particularly susceptible to these attacks, but anyone can have an intense anxiety attack under stress. Most of the time, these are situational and are less severe compared to panic attacks. Individuals may feel overwhelmed by the situation due to external or internal pressures and become extremely anxious. They generally build up over a period of time that can be minutes or hours, depending upon the situation. They usually are aware of what is going on and typically seek help or reassurance. They can be reassured, at least to an extent and may calm down with help, as opposed to a panic attack which may appear to not be under any (psychological) control. A panic attack can also be precipitated by a situation, and sometimes it can be anticipated, but the patients generally feel a distinct loss of control over the symptoms.

Panic disorder is treated with antidepressants such as SSRIs and psychotherapy. Cognitive behavioral therapy helps a lot as well. Benzodiazepines are very helpful in relieving and preventing anxiety symptoms but should be used with caution because they are habit-forming. Patients easily gravitate towards the pill as it gives immediate and predictable relief. However, in the long run, a lot of patients who take benzodiazepines like clonazepam or alprazolam become psychologically and physiologically dependent on them, and when they cannot have it, they become very anxious, partly because of the medication withdrawal and partly because of the fear of an anxiety attack. In general, daily use, especially with an escalating dose, should be avoided at any cost. Propranolol is a good option for symptom control.

An organic cause for the panic such as drug use, drug withdrawal, pheochromocytoma, migraine, hyperthyroidism, or other hormonal conditions should be ruled out. Sometimes, a brain tumor in the temporal lobe may present as panic attacks.

Quite often, patients with organic causes of panic attacks (and so other symptoms) alienate themselves from the symptoms as opposed to incorporating them into their lives. In other words, this can be explained as ego-dystonic as opposed to ego-syntonic. Ego-dystonic means the patient is aware of the symptoms and is bothered by them, and ego-syntonic means that the patient believes in the symptoms and incorporates in his or her thinking. They may not see the symptom as a problem because they incorporate the fear into themselves, i.e., their ego. A person with ego-syntonic symptoms (say, delusions) would claim that they are (certainly) being followed as opposed to ego-dystonic, where they would say "I have the thought that I am being followed." In case of panic attacks, a patient with a brain tumor might say, "I get these anxiety attacks, but I don't know why. I am sure there is something wrong with my head," which is ego-dystonic as opposed to "I am doomed, I am afraid something really bad is going to happen to me," which is ego-syntonic. Remember, this is not a hard and fast rule, but it should give an indication to make sure that we do not miss some organic cause. Even patients with organic causes of anxiety "learn" over a period of time to incorporate these symptoms into their lives, and patients with panic disorder learn to expect, manage, and even distance themselves from the symptoms in an intelligent manner. Interestingly, those patients who have a seizure or tumor causing the panic attack, feel relieved to find a cause of their suffering.

Agoraphobia

Agora in Greek means a gathering place or market, and agoraphobia is a fear of (being in) public places or situations where the patient may feel trapped, helpless, or embarrassed. Patients are afraid of not being able to "escape" from an uncomfortable situation. They keep thinking to themselves, "just in case, what if something happens to me and I need to make sure I escape?" The theme of not being able to escape or the potential for embarrassment may extend to any public place. What is mundane for most of us becomes destabilizing for these poor souls. It takes a considerable amount of effort for them to accomplish things that we all take for granted.

They might develop this fear after one or two panic attacks - essentially making them think, "What if I get a panic attack while I am on a train?", "What if I cannot breathe in a ballroom with a thousand people or what if I embarrass myself in front of the salesclerk?" "What if I get an anxiety attack and everyone thinks that I am going to get a heart attack, but it is truly a meaningless fear? What if they all come to know that I am mentally ill and unstable?"

Panic disorder and agoraphobia used to be linked together as panic disorder with and without agoraphobia as they occur together frequently, but the recent DSM delinked it because they can happen independently. The fear of going out in public, known as agoraphobia, might start after a panic attack but can become a problem of its own.

The fear may provoke significant anxiety to the point where the patient avoids all these places, and at times, confine themselves to a room. Even coming out of the house may be nerve-wracking. Although this fear of embarrassment and mild anxiety may be common among a lot of us, we can generally overcome it, and for a diagnosis of agoraphobia, the symptoms need to be severe, last for more than six months, and cause significant impairment to their lives. The fear should not be related to any other medical or psychological or drug problems.

Social Anxiety Disorder (Social Phobia)

This is a common condition, and it is estimated that about one out of 15 suffers from this. Unless you are a seasoned politician or one of the rare people who have Williams Syndrome[2], you might feel anxious or a

[2] Williams Syndrome is a genetic disorder resulting from the deletion of about 26 genes in chromosome 7. Affected people have specific facial features, heart and kidney problems, learning difficulties, and neurodevelopmental problems, among others. Interestingly they are exceedingly social and friendly. They would readily talk to any stranger

bit uncomfortable in most social settings. We all feel a bit of apprehension to meet strangers or important people or to be in a social situation that is not seen as very friendly or forgiving, such as office parties (as opposed to having dinner with the immediate family). We all fear being judged or fear that we might embarrass ourselves in the presence of strangers.

Our society is well aware of social anxiety (but not the disorder yet) and its potential to prevent people from living up to their potential. Every one of us can recall a situation where we were a bit too shy to ask that girl out or volunteer for an opportunity that could have changed our lives. Our societies have invented many formal gatherings, rules, and games that force us out of the shell of social anxiety. Every culture uses many excuses, from weddings to birthdays, and has devised methods to celebrate religious or cultural functions that incorporate social gatherings. Of course, our culture also invented alcohol, sometimes referred to as social lubricant, to help us glide through difficult social situations.

But unfortunately, for those who suffer from social anxiety disorder, these simple, joyful social situations can become living nightmares. These individuals dread any form of social interaction with unfamiliar people and have exaggerated fears of being negatively judged and scrutinized. They fear that they might do or say something that may embarrass or humiliate them. Social situations and anticipation of social situations cause significant anxiety and fear in these individuals to a point where they avoid social situations altogether, despite the desire to be social and the realization that their fear is irrational.

Social anxiety disorder typically starts at a young age, usually in teen years, with 80% of patients experiencing symptoms before age 20. The diagnostic criteria require 6 months of significant symptoms that interfere with day-to-day life. This disorder can be treated with SSRIs, anxiolytics, and behavioral therapy. When treated early, social anxiety disorder has a good prognosis, but like any anxiety disorder, the longer the patient suffers from it is harder to treat, as there is a major component of learning in the symptomatology of anxiety disorders.

Separation Anxiety Disorder

As the name implies, the core feature of this illness is an excessive, unbearable, and crippling distress with anxiety and fear in the context of separation from home or a caregiver like a mother. Separation anxi-

---

with sincere affection and friendliness in any setting. They typically light up any social situation. They also have a heightened sense of sound and are passionate about music. Here is a footnote to a footnote: People with Down's syndrome (extra chromosome in 21) also are rather very social and like music.

ety is part of natural development in children below age three. But, the patients with separation anxiety disorder, who are also mostly children, but older than three, excessively worry when separated, or in anticipation of separation from home or a loved one, to the point that their day-to-day functioning becomes impaired. A lot of these kids cannot even go to school because they feel extremely anxious while they are away from home. They worry and fear that something terrible or catastrophic might happen to the caretaker or themselves (mom might have a heart attack and die, or I might get lost or kidnapped or die alone). They refuse to go to school, refuse to stay alone - even at home, and refuse to sleep outside of home. They may get nightmares, and quite often, young kids complain of various physical symptoms (tummy ache) when put in these situations.

Most of the kids grow out of this with or without treatment, but when this is present, it can be a significant impediment for the child's progress. Cognitive behavioral therapy focused on identifying the anxiety-provoking situations, and slowly exposing and desensitizing the child help them come out of this problem. Some of them may need anti-anxiety medications or antidepressants. In general, these children grow out of this, but they seem to develop anxiety disorders such as social anxiety or panic attacks later in life. Alcoholism is also more prevalent with people who have anxiety issues.

Interestingly, anxiety disorders run in families and children with separation anxiety may have adults with an anxiety disorder in the family. In addition to the genetic contribution, an anxious mother can make the child anxious. This needs to be kept in mind when treating a child because quite often, the adult caregiver may also need help - if not to reduce their own anxiety -but to help them help their children.

Specific Phobias, or Phobias

A lot of us may have some fear or discomfort over a thing or two (snakes, spiders) in life, but we generally are fine and go about our lives by avoiding those. For example, very few people are comfortable or unafraid of snakes, but most of us are fine because it is not something we need to deal with on a day-to-day basis (thank god for that!)[3]. While I might not choose to live in or near a snake park, I am going to be fine if I stay away from them. The snake or the thought of snakes may not bother me much, so my life may not be affected much. Similarly, if someone

---

3 There was a movie named Snakes on a Plane. The trailer says this "Imagine your worst fears. The ones that paralyze you. The ones that render you helpless. Now imagine them all at once" in a bragging tone trying to sell the movie, which in essence, is a pain for a lot of people.

is afraid of driving, they might get by with public transportation or a driver, and it may be an inconvenience but not a disorder - yet.

But when these kinds of fears interfere with life, it becomes a problem. Patients with a phobia are severely affected by the object of their phobia, be it snake, flying, bridges, clowns, spider, or thunder. The key difference from normal fear and a diagnosable phobia is the degree of discomfort and impairment or how much it affects their lives. For example, even a picture of a snake, or thought, or even a mention of the word "snake" can freeze some of these patients with a phobia of snakes. This intense fear or phobia may affect their day to day life, and they might constantly worry about coming across a snake in even the most unlikely places or times. When the phobia is of something, we need to do on a day-to-day basis like driving or flying, it becomes more interfering and disabling.

Phobias often develop because the patients learn by association of a scary event that happened in the past. The treatment of phobia is essentially breaking the association through slow exposure to the object. For example, someone who is afraid of snakes will be exposed to a snake little by little, starting with a simple drawing and then progress to pictures. The patient will observe these until the fear is gone, and actually, they might get bored looking at them. Then, they can see the snake from a distance, play with toys that look like a snake, and move on to touch and play with real snakes. Some patients may need SSRIs and anxiolytics. It is important to keep in mind that people with a phobia may have other anxiety disorders, depression, or alcohol use as these disorders are common in patients as well as in family members.

Obsessive-Compulsive Disorder (OCD)

If there is one illness, we all can relate to and easily understand its symptoms (but of course not the illness), it is OCD. We all go through times in our lives when we may have obsessive thoughts and compulsive behaviors, especially under stress. On occasions, we may have worried about leaving the stove on or leaving the iron on or the car unlocked, which caused discomfort or anxiety. Similarly, we may have knocked on wood or uttered a small prayer to avert something bad - imagined or real - happening. Although they are not obsessions, compulsions, or OCD, the same idea or psychological mechanism is at play in OCD, only in a tremendously painful manner.

Obsessions

Obsessions are unintended intrusive thoughts (which can be an image or impulse) that keep coming to the mind, causing significant discomfort and anxiety. For example, a patient may constantly worry about germs in his hands that he knows he does not have, and he has no need to worry about, but can't stop. He may wash his hands to get rid of the worry (not necessarily the germs), knowing fully well that he does not need to wash them. He may feel better for a while after washing, but the thought persists, continuing to knock on the brain's door, annoyingly regularly and intensifying as he tries to ignore it. He might wash once, twice, or numerous times a day, but the worry continues since the actual issue is not the cleanliness. The intrusive thoughts can be aggressive (fear of harming someone), contamination, sexual (forbidden or perverse thoughts), somatic, cleaning, checking, and repeating (rewriting or writing over and over).

Although the patients know that these obsessions are unrealistic and meaningless, they cannot suppress or ignore them. Instead, they spend all day thinking about it. It is important to note that the patients with OCD typically know that the thoughts are not real, although on rare occasions, they may lose insight and start believing it. In psychosis, the patient typically loses insight, meaning that they fully believe in their delusions, even when it is not plausible (like, there is a transmitter in my tooth that records what I think)[4]. The obsessions are seen as meaningless, annoying and intrusive thoughts, which might actually increase anxiety by making them feel bad about having these irrational thoughts.

Some common obsessions
• Contamination: Fear about body fluids, germs, or chemicals and radiation
• Harming: Fear of harming others or causing damage, loss of control resulting in harm to others.
• Sexual thoughts: Forbidden sexual images, acts, or thoughts
• Being perfect: Organization of things or events.
• Being religious or pious: Thinking bad thoughts about god, offending god

While feeling petrified and guilty, patients try hard to ignore or suppress the obsessions, only to see them persist tenaciously or come back with a vengeance. They resort to performing rituals, some of them equally meaningless, to reduce the anxiety and mitigate the distress. These rituals may reduce the anxiety for the moment, but they actually reinforce the behavior, and the obsessions always come back, leading them to do increasingly more elaborate rituals. For example, washing hands might make a patient feel better about the germs on his hands for a short while, but the worry, doubt, or obsession comes back, and they become more intent on doing a better job of washing. The next wash, they try harder or wash more than once, just to make sure the worries do not come back again, but soon they start doubting the quality of the wash and then go back to wash again, then again, and again, repeatedly all day, every day. Sometimes these rituals become elaborate, methodical, and time consuming.

Compulsions

Compulsions are actions that one does to make the obsessions, or the anxiety caused by obsessions, go away. They sometimes are related to the compulsions and make "sense," like washing hands with the fear of germs, but sometimes they do not make sense, like avoiding walking on the lines of the pavement to avert cancer. These compulsions can be thoughts like a prayer or even images, for example, a mental image of god to counter a bad thought. These behaviors typically do not have a purpose other than to reduce anxiety caused by obsession or an attempt to suppress the obsessions. The ritualistic behavior of a religiously preoccupied man or an elaborate ritual of a superstitious athlete are not compulsions, even though these are done to reduce anxiety. It is one thing to pack your athletic bag in a certain way as a good luck charm, but it is completely different to be preoccupied with the contents of the bag all day every day.

The most well-known example is "germaphobia," where a person worries nonstop about getting germs on their hands and washing their hands. Some of us might be very particular about the way we wash our hands or keeping things clean. A person who is a "clean freak" but who does not have OCD may worry about the dirt on their hands even to a point of distress and may go to the bathroom to scrub their hands often, especially when they touch something dirty. They may even be ritualistic in their hand-washing, but they are typically satisfied and resume normal activities. What differentiates those with OCD is that the person with OCD will NOT be satisfied after washing and they go back to wash again. They won't ever be satisfied even after numerous washes, even when they sincerely believe and clearly know that they do not even need to wash in the first place. The preoccupation with the obsessions, the consequential anxiety, as well as the resulting compulsive behavior often consumes the patient's entire day.

There are several conditions that present with symptoms similar to OCD as described below.

Obsessive Compulsive Personality Disorder or OCPD

The main difference of OCPD from OCD is that the patient with OCPD does not describe intrusive, unwanted, or irrational thoughts. They believe their thoughts about being tidy clean and organized are rational and meaningful. They are perfectionists and want to be perfectionists. They feel anxious if they are not organized, but do not feel the anxiety is a bad thing. They know that they are different but are not worried that they are "crazy," and they may be proud of being organized and get annoyed by others who are not. While they spend time and effort in being organized, they do not spend excessive time on quelling the anxiety and distress of the obsessions.

Autism Spectrum Disorders

Patients with autism sometimes exhibit ritualistic behavior, but unlike OCD, they do not perform the ritual for a specific purpose (of reducing anxiety from an obsession). For example, patients with autism may do something specific for no apparent purpose, such as taking a walk in a certain manner, through a certain path, every single day. They may get agitated if they cannot do it, but once they do, they forget about it. Similarly, they may keep things in their room in a specific order (with no apparent internal or external reason), and when the order is disrupted, they get upset, but once the order is restored, they do not worry about it. For example, a person with autism may have an "obsessive" interest in superman action figures, and they may collect hundreds of them. They may arrange these figures in an order, which may not be obvious for the rest of us. They would know if someone altered it and may get upset. They would rearrange everything, but not worry about it after they rearrange once. A person with OCD may have an internal reason for maintaining the order. Quite often, autistic rituals do not seem to have any reason or motivation behind the orderliness.

PANDAS

Pediatric Autoimmune Neuropsychiatric Disorders Associated with Streptococcal Infections or Pediatric Acute Onset Neuropsychiatric Syndrome, or PANDAS or PANS. This is an intriguing disease that exemplifies the intersection between biology and psychology - here, a bacterial infection, an autoimmune response, and the brain.

Thomas Szasz wrote a book titled "Myth of Mental Illness," which claimed that mental illnesses are invented by the psychiatrists to make a living. This statement was mockingly quoted in the book "Epigenetics of Schizophrenia" by Irving Gottesman, claiming, "If schizophrenia is a myth, it is a myth with a genetic component." In that vein, PANDAS can be called a myth with an autoimmune component.

Streptococcus is a fascinating bacterium that is present in the skin and throat. It causes the throat infection called strep throat and skin infection called Impetigo. The bacteria have an interesting cover composed of a molecule that is very similar to the one in the interstitial connective tissue of the human heart, joints, kidney, and brain. This concept is called Molecular Mimicry. The bacteria have an advantage in avoiding an immune response as it mimics a natural molecule. But unfortunately, this can go wrong, and after an acute infection, the body may produce antibodies against the shared molecule. These antibodies then erroneously attack the heart, joint, or brain cells causing rheumatic fever which can affect the heart, skin, joints, and brain.

When the brain is involved, it frequently causes a movement disorder known as Sydenham's chorea, in which patients have choreatic movements of hands, legs, and sometimes facial muscles and tongue. Unlike Parkinson's disease, they are non-rhythmic, uncoordinated, jerky, flailing movements that look like a bad dance[5], and the patients try to mask it by doing something like wiping the face. Hence it is called semi-purposive movement. These can occur within six months of the rheumatic fever and typically start abruptly.

Similarly, the patients afflicted with a strep infection and rheumatic fever can also develop OCD, which might look very similar to conventional OCD. However, these patients have a very abrupt onset of the illness, typically within a day. Besides being associated with the infection and abrupt onset or abrupt change in the intensity of symptoms, they may also have neurological symptoms like abnormal movements, anxiety and anxiety attacks, and vocal or motor tics. The treatment of this OCD is similar to treating regular OCD with SSRIs and CBT, in addition to the treatment of the streptococcal infection and the acute rheumatic fever. However, these patients do not tolerate the SSRIs well, so the medicine needs to be started at a very low dose and increased slowly.

There are few other conditions that confuse OCD. People with impulse control disorders such as compulsive gambling or addictions may have intense preoccupation about the next "fix," but these are not considered obsessions as they are not irrational or unwanted in the same sense as obsessions.

People with body dysmorphic disorder are severely preoccupied by an imagined or exaggerated abnormality of their body, such as a crooked nose, and may spend all their time worrying about it or trying to fix it. This is not OCD, although it may be very difficult to understand or differentiate. They are usually preoccupied about just one thing in their

---

5 Chorea in Greek means dance. Same etymology as choreography. This condition is also called St. Vitus Dance.

body and usually believe that they have a deformity. Unlike OCD, these patients do not consider that their belief is irrational. Their belief may be so strong, at times appearing delusional. They also do not do things to improve their condition magically, but instead might get a plastic surgery. They may not be satisfied even after the surgery, which makes it difficult to understand this illness and differentiate it from OCD.

Body Focused Repetitive Behaviors

The classic example of Body Focused Repetitive Behaviors is Trichotillomania, or habitual hair pulling. Again, in this condition, there are no obsessions or intrusive thoughts, and the thought and behavior lack the typical (magical) cause-and-effect of OCD.

Hoarding

Hoarding behavior used to be considered as a type of OCD, but a typical hoarder believes that they need, or may need, at some point, the things they collect - be it an old newspaper or used packaging material. They may recognize that it is excessive but are not typically bothered by their behavior.

Patients with Tic Disorder might exhibit repetitive behavior that generally brings a lot of stress. The behavior is not only unwanted, but a distinct difference to be noted is the fact that these behaviors do not have full control like in rituals of OCD.

Schizophrenia and OCD are a bit more complex. It appears that they co-occur, meaning OCD symptoms are found often in schizophrenia. It is unclear whether this OCD is similar to stereotypical OCD. Obsessions and compulsions can occur transiently or longer in patients with other illnesses like depression, and GAD. Patients with typical OCD know their thoughts are meaningless and irrational, but the DSM-5 has the option of OCD with poor insight, meaning that they may not realize their thoughts are irrational. Patients with schizophrenia who have delusions sometimes have good insight. This can get confusing both while learning about it and occasionally while seeing patients. It is important to remember to try to understand it from the patient's point of view and assess the symptom in a psychological and conceptual way, which will help understand the symptoms better. For example, patients with developmental disability may have odd preoccupations and repetitive behaviors. They are sometimes diagnosed with OCD, but they do not have the intrusiveness and anxiety of obsessions, and they readily admit that their preoccupation is intentional and not bothersome.

Treatment of Anxiety disorders

The treatment of anxiety disorders constitute antidepressants, anxiolytics, and behavior therapy. Overall, anxiety disorders are easy to diagnose and treat, and it is one of those conditions that is rewarding for the clinician to see the patients improve dramatically. However, at times, these may prove to be a challenge to treat, especially among the patients with chronic anxiety disorders. Some of them may "worry too much" about everything and hesitate to venture into taking medications or engaging in therapy. Even when the illness is adequately treated, or even when the symptoms are under control, some patients may continue to worry, which may or may not be a problem. There is a large learning component to the fear and anxiety, and so even if the medications work well, they need behavioral therapy, and it typically takes months for the patients to get better.

Antidepressants

The first line of treatment in any anxiety disorder is an antidepressant and SSRIs (fluoxetine, paroxetine, sertraline, and citalopram) are the most popular because they are very effective and easy to administer, have minimal side effects, and rarely need a dose adjustment. Other antidepressants like tricyclics and other newer SNRIs (venlafaxine or duloxetine) also work well. Bupropion works differently and also helps in anxiety, but it is not the first choice for many doctors because it has a stimulant effect and some patients with anxiety feel uncomfortable taking it, especially at the beginning.

Clomipramine was the first drug to be approved for OCD, so there is some preference of clomipramine for OCD, but no evidence exists suggesting its superiority over other tricyclics medications such as imipramine or amitriptyline. However, it is common for patients with OCD to be prescribed clomipramine over other medications. These days SSRIs are the primary medications for OCD, other anxiety disorders, as well as depression. SSRIs have become some of the most ubiquitously used medications like statins or acid reducers because of their relative safety and ease of use. I always advise my non-psychiatrist colleagues to use SSRIs when they are in doubt.

Similarly, buspirone was initially approved for anxiety disorder and was heavily marketed as an anti-anxiety drug. While it is an effective drug, it needs to be taken several times a day and dosing needs some adjustment. It has not been proven to be superior to SSRIs, which are administered once a day and the dosing may be simpler. Fluvoxamine is another medication that has special status as it was approved for OCD initially, but clinicians generally prefer popular SSRIs like fluoxetine, paroxetine, or citalopram as their first choice over fluvoxamine.

Anxiolytics

Benzodiazepines are highly addictive, but they are excellent medications that can offer immediate, effective, and even pleasant relief from anxiety. Diazepam (Valium), lorazepam (Ativan), clonazepam (Klonopin), and alprazolam (Xanax) are some of the most commonly used and abused drugs in the world. They all have street value and are frequently abused. However, they are highly effective medications sometimes not chosen by physicians due to the potential for addiction, abuse, and tolerance issues of the drug. They are excellent medications in acute settings but are problematic to use them long term. There are clear situations where these benzodiazepines should and should not be used, as follows:

Appropriate Use of Benzodiazepines
• Initial treatment period. When a patient is diagnosed for the first time, they can take these with clear knowledge of the addiction potential until the SSRIs and CBT take effect. A simple rule of thumb is that they can take them daily for no more than two weeks.
• As needed use – do not exceed one or two pills a week in the long term.
• Low fixed dose daily, even with occasional "PRN" use is accepted as long as patients do not escalate in the dosing. Some patients take 5mg of diazepam for 20 years and benefit from anxiety control. Even among these patients, it may be argued that they have become tolerant and dependent on the medication, and it is not therapeutic. Chronic use can actually cause rebound or withdrawal anxiety.
Unacceptable use:
• Dose escalation: increasing the dose to gain the same effect is tolerance.
• Dependence: not feeling normal without the benzodiazepines or excessive anxiety - psychological or physiological distress in the absence or anticipated absence of the benzodiazepines is called dependence.
• High dose: it is physiologically unacceptable for anyone to be on a high dose of benzodiazepines such as 8mg of clonazepam a day. They are essentially tackling the dependence.

Quite often, when educated about the addiction potential, patients (at least most of them) generally hesitate to take them, or as to their nature, "worry" about getting addicted. Patients with problems such as dependence or addiction are the ones who argue, cajole, or convince the prescribers to give them these. Any patient who gets a high dose of benzodiazepines month after month should be evaluated for addiction and dependence.

Non-benzodiazepine anxiolytics

Propranolol: Propranolol is a beta-blocker that slows the heart and nullifies the effects of adrenaline. Adrenaline mediates all the symptoms of anxiety including increased heart rate, high blood pressure, etc that feed into more anxiety. Propranolol, by blocking these effects sends a message of calm to the brain, and so, reduces the anxiety without clouding the mind. Propranolol also blocks the central effects of norepinephrine (adrenaline) and is believed to suppress the memory formation involved in the origins of PTSD (see next chapter) and so seems to have a prophylactic effect on PTSD.

Gabapentin (Neurontin) has become a very popular non-benzodiazepine medication in the treatment of anxiety disorders. Gabapentin was synthesized to mimic the inhibitory neurotransmitter GABA, which plays a major role in anxiety. Gabapentin does have addiction potential, but it is a relatively safe drug with a very high therapeutic range (from 100 mg to 3600 mg a day). Interestingly, this is one of the medications that has an inversely proportional bioavailability, meaning the more you take, the lower the percentage of it reaches the blood system (60% of 900 = 540 and 50% of 1200 = 600). Although it increases in general, it does not increase proportionally to the dose.

Hydroxyzine[6]: (Vistaril, Atarax) is an antihistamine that is widely used for anxiety control. It is sedating and can be used for sleep.

Melatonin: melatonin is a widely used supplement for insomnia. Some believe that this helps anxiety. While it is possible that by being a mild sedative, it can have calming effects, the direct evidence is not convincing.

Cognitive behavioral therapy

Cognitive behavioral therapy or psychotherapy (CBT) based on learning principles is widely used, scientifically proven, relatively more objective, and somewhat easier to administer than other forms of psychotherapies. CBT, in simple terms, is learning. We constantly learn to make our lives better, more comfortable, and less painful, whether it is

---

6 Apparently, this is the only word in English that has X, Y and Z in a row...

learning a new language, skill, or learning how to avoid problems. For example, when we first learn to drive or ride a bike, we are petrified to the extent that every car seems to come to crash on us and every tree seems to be right in the middle of the path. What if the fear gets you and you give up learning to drive? The fear will persist. Most of us have this fear but still practice enough to a point where we lose the fear. Here, the thought of crashing the car is somewhat irrational and the fear is excessive, which influences our behavior so that we would not practice, which may be detrimental. But we get over this by "exposing" ourselves to the danger until we master the technique.

The idea behind CBT is that the patients can learn to recognize the distortions in their thought, be trained to control their emotions and behavior, and thus improve their symptoms. There is a learning component for many of the symptoms, and so, the anxiety can be unlearned. The same idea goes behind the development and treatment of many psychiatric symptoms.

Desensitization is a method employed in anxiety treatment. This is done in a methodical step by step manner for each specific fear the patient has. The first step is to educate the patient about the nature of the illness and how the patients learn to be afraid. Then, they need help identifying the fears or anxiety provoking things or situations (going out in public, snakes, or dirt on their desk), and make a list.

The patients will be taught to monitor their anxiety and asked to give a score on their level of their anxiety. Then, they will gradually be exposed to these anxiety-provoking situations very slowly, starting from the least threatening to the most threatening situation.

For example, in the case of snake phobia, one can start with a friendly cartoon of a snake, then a picture of a real snake, and later on, an actual snake. The patients may feel extreme anxiety even when they see the cartoon at first, but the way the therapy works is that the patient would continue looking at the picture until the anxiety dissipates. Once they feel comfortable with the cartoon, they can move on to looking at a real picture until they lose the fear of that picture, and so on. While they do this, they would start with a therapist or a family member next to them for support to handle the anxiety, but they will also slowly wean off of the need to have someone with them for safety.

Applying the same principles, fearful situations like public speaking, going out in public, traveling on a plane, or driving over a bridge can be mastered step by step. Flooding is a technique where you would put the patient in a room with one hundred snakes and leave the patient alone until he or she loses the fear. I am not sure if I would volunteer for this, but it seems to work occasionally. This is a not popular method of treatment, as it can be destabilizing.

Quite often, patients may need to take a course of medication and get stabilized before going in for therapy. The patients may also use anxiolytics initially, such as benzodiazepines or propranolol, when they are "exposed." It is important to note that some patients actually feel worse during the exposure, but they need to persist and stay with the treatment until they get better. The idea is to persist until the anxiety subsides every time they sit for an exposure session. In some patients with PTSD, the exposure can worsen the illness, and so it should be used with caution.

Comorbidity and complications

Comorbidity or occurrence of one psychiatric illness with another one is very common. About half of the patients diagnosed with one illness also have another one. Anxiety disorders, alcoholism, and depression seem to occur together in the same person or in the same families, implying a genetic cause. Anxiety is a common symptom in several mental illnesses, including psychosis and PTSD. Patients with anxiety are prone to alcoholism because of the calming effects of alcohol, and many patients describe that alcohol makes them feel "normal." They are also likely to become dependent or addicted to benzodiazepines. Comorbidity makes it difficult to treat patients.

Without knowing the exact pathophysiology of these illnesses, one can only speculate on the possible reasons of such comorbidity. The diagnostic overlap of symptomatology between diagnostic categories, biological, or etiological overlap may possibly contribute to the comorbidity. However, comorbidity or overlapping symptoms and diagnoses is an important clinical issue to keep in mind when approaching a patient with anxiety or any other symptoms.

Neuroticism

Neuroticism is a personality trait often characterized in colloquial usage as excessive worry or concern for orderliness. People considered highly neurotic are seen to worry about mundane things, anxious all the time, and get frustrated easily, especially when things do not go the way they want or when there are surprises. When neuroticism is measured, it follows a bell curve or a "normal distribution" with the majority of us in the middle with a score around the average, with a few scoring on the high and low ends, like many biological or psychological attributes. People who score high on the neuroticism scale seem to be more susceptible to anxiety disorders. High neuroticism may be biologically associated with anxiety disorders, but it is unclear whether there is any

Anxiety Disorders

causal relationship between the two. Anything in excess is not healthy, and so is worrying. At the same time, not worrying or very low neuroticism may also be harmful.

Chapter 8

PTSD and Trauma Related Disorders

Trauma, by definition, is an unsettling and disturbing experience. It permanently changes the core of the person and stays in their memory for the rest of their life. Someone who witnesses a gruesome murder may not look at life or other human beings in the same manner again, and a victim of sexual abuse may not be able to have the same perspective about love and sex again.

Trauma takes away the innocence and impairs the victim's ability to trust. For the victim, the world is not benign, safe, and predictable anymore, and instead, it becomes predatory and threatening. The experience of trauma changes one's perspective by taking away the joy and replacing it with a painful suspicion and distrust.

Although every traumatic experience can be harmful and damaging, not everyone who goes through trauma develops PTSD. Even the harmful effect or loss of innocence can be argued as a component of growing up. In fact, many children who experience trauma, especially at the societal level such as war or natural disaster, emerge unscathed and lead successful lives. However, a lot of us suffer lifelong maladjustment following a destabilizing trauma. Trauma is unfortunate but PTSD is cruel.

PTSD

PTSD is a morbid and pathological adjustment or reaction to the trauma that haunts and cripples the patient. Like any mental illness, PTSD or response to trauma varies in severity ranging from some becoming well-adjusted and successful after the trauma with a quiet sadness underneath, or just a lingering disappointment about the loss, to a total disability. For example, refugees and migrants may have recurring memories and dreams of their lost land and life which may not meet the criteria for PTSD, and they might eventually become well-adjusted to the new life and may become very successful. But, when they develop PTSD, they may end up living a meaningless, monotonous existence filled with pain and sorrow.

Diagnosis

The diagnosis of PTSD using the DSM has become a bit more specific and detailed with the changes in the DSM 5. These include five components: 1) a history of trauma, 2) re-experiencing of the trauma like flashbacks or ruminations, 3) avoidance of triggers like people, situations or thoughts and feelings that remind the person of the trauma, 4) severe emotional reaction such as depression, suspicion or distortion of the memory, and 5) hyperarousal or hypervigilance especially associated with the triggers.

The DSM criteria specify trauma as a threat to life or sexual violence that is experienced, witnessed, learned, or seen at work, like among first responders. Although trauma that leads to a PTSD is usually quite morbid, sometimes what seems to be a mundane thing like being rear-ended in a car, failing an exam, a major embarrassment, or severe emotional injuries such as the betrayal of infidelity can lead to PTSD.

The most bothersome symptom of PTSD is the recurring memory of the trauma that is intrusive, unwanted, and unpleasant. These memories are loaded with fear and pain and pop into their heads randomly for no apparent reason. The patients may ruminate about the trauma and dwell in the past, although it is unpleasant and generally evokes negative emotions of pain, sadness, suspicion, and anger. A bystander may say, "forget about it and move on," but these memories come upon without control and torment them. Unlike obsessions, these are not seen as irrational or meaningless by the patient, and instead, they fear these thoughts because they bring upon intense psychological and physiological distress.

An extreme form of this is called a flashback, in which the patient essentially relives the experience. During a flashback, patients are generally aware that it is not real, but they cognitively and emotionally respond as if they are back in the same traumatic situation with the same level or more fear. Sometimes this can become a dissociative state where the patient may not be fully aware of the present surroundings. Dreams and nightmares of the trauma also have a similar distressing effect.

Although these memories and flashbacks can occur anytime for no reason, quite often they are precipitated by a reminder or a trigger. Witnessing a similar event of the trauma or seeing a person who reminds them of the perpetrator, smell, lighting, or words of the trauma, all can trigger a memory or a flashback. They avoid the triggers that cause anger, depression, or anxiety. Unfortunately, when they feel angry, depressed, or anxious for unrelated reasons, these feelings can also act as triggers. The mind gets trained in a loop; every time they face a trigger, it brings back memories that make them sad and angry, and conversely, the sadness and anger from unrelated events can bring back the memories of the trauma.

So, they avoid the triggers, both external and internal. External triggers include people or places that remind them of the trauma, and internal triggers include the memory, thought or even the feeling associated with the trauma. Smell related to the trauma seems to be a significant trigger that brings back memories and emotions of the trauma. It is cyclical. The patient may think about the trauma, feel particularly depressed about it, which makes them have a flashback and worsens the depression which in turn, as a negative affect associated with the memory of the trauma, can bring back the memory. Sometimes patients with PTSD get worse as they suffer more, or even when they try to get help by talking about the trauma, it triggers the memory, and so on.

This cycle alters the cognition and mood of the patient significantly. They start thinking that the world is dangerous and that no one can be trusted. They feel bad about themselves and their past and have a negative outlook about their future. One of the most famous examples of this is known as "survivor guilt," in which the patient who survived the trauma when someone else died, like in combat, feels bad that it is him or her who should have died not the friend. This can be intense when the other person dies trying to save the patient. They may think in negative terms about themselves with fear, anger, or guilt. In addition, they may become reclusive and disengage from social activities because they do not trust or enjoy any positive emotions. Sometimes, they shut down and do not remember the traumatic event or the details surrounding it. Frequently, patients may appear to function alright outwardly, but they may detach themselves emotionally and cognitively with no interest in participating in life. They simply exist and do not live.

On the other hand, some patients experience marked alteration in the arousal, a classic example of which is known as hypervigilance, where the patients are in a state of heightened awareness of fear and anxiety. They show an exaggerated startle response. They may get angry easily, behave recklessly, involve themselves in self-destructive or threatening behavior, and get into fights. Often, they fail in their responsibilities and lose focus and confidence. While they may be daring and dangerous on the one hand, they may not take any acceptable risks like taking responsibility at work or with their families because of a lack of confidence about themselves and mistrust of society. They have sleep problems and may use drugs and alcohol excessively.

Treatment

PTSD has no specific treatment. There is no particular medication that is proven to help patients with PTSD. However, numerous medications are clinically used with varying degrees of anecdotal success, especially for symptomatic treatment for depression or anxiety. Usually, the clinicians approach the patient to address the symptoms specifically with a large degree of support, understanding, and acceptance. Patients who have alcohol or drug abuse benefit from treatment for substance use. Antidepressants such as SSRIs seem to help patients with PTSD - with or without symptoms of depression. Anti-anxiety medications also help individuals with hyperarousal-related symptoms. Antipsychotics and mood stabilizers are used with varying degrees of anecdotal success. Prazosin, an alpha-adrenergic agonist at 1 or 2 mg taken at night, seems to help patients with severe nightmares.

Usually, when you come across someone with severe PTSD, they may have tried one or all of these medications or are taking several of these. At times, it seems that while none of the medications work, the patients choose to take something strong and sedating to numb the symptoms. Benzodiazepines, which are highly addictive or habit-forming, are frequently preferred and abused by some of these patients. Some even prefer antipsychotics for the calming effect. Considering the high prevalence of addiction and the high propensity of dependence among these patients who suffer unbearable anxiety, depression, and psychic pain, the clinician is often placed in a dilemma about the choice of medications. It is hard to watch these patients suffer while refusing to provide comforting medications, especially when you see that the patients are addicted or dependent. It is a lose-lose predicament.

Similarly, psychotherapy for PTSD seems to lack clarity in terms of techniques and benefit. For example, psychological debriefing after the trauma seems to follow the intuitive principles of letting things out or clearing one's mind so that the memory does not stay there and haunt for life. This would be expected to prevent PTSD in the future but does not seem to have the purported benefit. In fact, it might worsen or increase the chances of PTSD by kindling the effect or reinforcing the memory and their outlook of the event. In the same way, some patients say that therapy and talking about the trauma triggers them to have PTSD symptoms and makes the illness worse, at least initially.

However, in general, support, understanding, and expression or care through listening and being there helps. Psycho-education helps patients understand the illness. Helping patients separate the traumatic memory and the negative emotions leads to good symptomatic improvement, but it is easier said than done.

Besides support, proven method of psychotherapy is CBT. CBT, like in anxiety, involves exposure and desensitization. However, this does have a danger of kindling the memories, triggering the flashbacks, and thus worsening the illness. Care must be employed to not expose the patient to too much too soon. The idea of CBT is to separate the memories from the emotions, but when the emotion itself is the memory, it is hard to work with. Yet, a focus on the reduction of anxiety and relaxation would help the patient. As you can imagine, there is a significant component of learning and conditioning in the symptomatology of PTSD, and so one can be hopeful that some of these can be unlearned over a period of time. There is no clear or convincing evidence for other forms of therapy, but what patient wants or thinks as beneficial should be offered on a case by case basis. Some patients seem to benefit from group therapy, which includes patients who have experienced the same or similar trauma and exhibit similar symptoms. There is a camaraderie, understanding, and brotherhood among the survivors that is alien to others.

Other Trauma Related Illnesses

Acute Stress Disorder

Acute stress disorder is not an uncommon immediate response to a trauma in which the patient experiences intense negative emotions of shock, fear, depression, and avoidance behavior along with disinterest in daily activities. The illness occurs immediately after trauma (ranging from one day to one month). At times it appears to be very similar to PTSD, but it usually gets better after a month, with or without interventions. However, it can continue after a month and meet the criteria for PTSD. Acute stress disorder increases the probability of later PTSD. The principles of safety, support, and symptomatic treatment to reduce symptoms such as anxiety, insomnia, and depression should be employed. Using propranolol at this moment seem to help reduce anxiety and minimize the risk of future PTSD. This seems to work by interfering with the formation of a deep memory of the trauma leading to PTSD. Benzodiazepines may also work the same way. Interestingly, people who are drunk in an accident seem to have less incidence of PTSD than who are not drunk. Also, the soldiers who encountered trauma but received a shot of morphine are less likely to get PTSD.

Adjustment Disorder

Adjustment disorder is the emotional and behavioral problems that occur following trauma or stress and typically start after a month and last until six months (acute) or longer (chronic). The subtypes include adjustment disorder with depression, anxiety, conduct disorder, or mixed symptoms. Bereavement or adjustment disorder after bereavement has been introduced as a separate disorder known as persistent complex bereavement disorder.

Persistent Complex Bereavement Disorder

One of the frequently faced dilemmas for a clinician or a caregiver is dealing with someone who is grieving because quite often it is unclear when or whether they need intervention. Grief is one of the major life events that every one of us will experience at some point. It is painful and disruptive under any circumstances, although a normal grief reaction may not be considered a disease. There is no clear evidence of benefit from any kind of intervention in normal grief. Individuals who go through normal grief may benefit from emotional support or supportive therapy and experience a reduction of symptoms immediately, but they seem to do well in the long run with or without such intervention. Some even argue against the intervention of the normal and natural grief process. Some patients might hesitate to accept help because they feel that it is equivalent to being unfaithful to the person they just lost.

But there are a lot of individuals who might seek help or advice, and some of them may have significant symptoms or disruptions of their routine and may need a bit of direction. On the one hand, it may seem obvious or intuitive to help a patient who is seeking help, which may make it easier to determine the need for psychotherapy and support. Cultures around the world have elaborate rituals around death and loss to support the grieving and help them recover to normal life and to reduce the pain of loss. However, severe or complex or prolonged grief can be detrimental and may need intervention.

In fact, research has shown that in cases of complicated grief or prolonged and severe grief, the evidence for the benefit of an intervention is clear. So, it is important to understand, identify and address the pathological grief, now named as Persistent Complex Bereavement Disorder (PCBD). Although debatable, normal grief includes feelings of loss and yearning for the lost one, sadness, and depression - known here as sorrow, avoidance of reminders of the lost one, a preoccupation of the death and circumstances of death, self-blame, shock and denial of the loss, isolation from others, and avoidance of pleasurable activities. These vary in intensity and duration but, in general, people get better

PTSD and Trauma Related Disorders

with all these emotions, thoughts, and experiences in a few weeks to months. It is a problem if they do not get better or get worse.

Of note here are the famous 5 stages of loss or grief by Elizabeth Kubler Ross, including Shock and Denial, Anger, Bargaining, Depression and Acceptance, is an interesting and popular way to describe any loss. There are several theories describing grief, but many people experience the symptoms described above. Some healthy people do recover from the loss quickly - within a few days - and move on with routine things in life.

The essential features of Persistent Complex Bereavement Disorder are similar to normal grief but are more intense and prolonged. These include an intense yearning and longing for the lost one, severe sorrow, emotional pain, and sadness that does not get better over a period of time and instead may get worse. The patient may be intensely preoccupied with the death of the loved one and the circumstances around the death, sometimes all day, every day without thinking about or doing anything else. They remain in shock and feel numb, lose their healthy feeling and normal emotions, refuse to accept the death, and continue to be bitter and angry about the loss. They avoid things that remind them of their lost one, refuse to reminisce about the dead in a positive manner, and have negative thoughts, including self-blame. They may feel lonely, choose to stay alone, become disinterested in socializing or interacting with others, often complaining that they cannot function without the dead one, they feel incomplete, and refuse to pursue interests or stop enjoying life.

A lot of people who grieve may show these symptoms. Society may be understanding and sympathetic towards the grieving - to a certain point. When this goes on for a long time, especially when it disrupts the survivor's life and when they fail to meet the needs and requirements of their day to day life, people start to worry or get annoyed. This may be the ideal time to offer help or intervene but may experience resistance from the patients.

There are two other illnesses included in this section of trauma-related illnesses, including Reactive Attachment Disorder and Disinhibited Social Engagement Disorder. These two occur in childhood and are related to neglect. In reactive attachment disorder (of childhood), the children have difficulty attaching to a caregiver. The children have difficulty in approaching or coming to an adult caregiver for comfort, protection, support, or nurturance, despite the children having the capacity and desire to form such an attachment. This was noted in abandoned babies of war and migration.

In Disinhibited Social Engagement disorder, children do not have normal reluctance or shyness in relating to strangers, and instead, they become overly familiar and have odd and meaningless attachments. This is also known to be related or resulting from neglect and poor care by the caregiver. These are relatively rare, and supportive therapy will help the children to improve.

Chapter 9

Eating Disorders

Eating disorders are not lifestyle choices or new food or dieting fads. These are serious illnesses that can even be life-threatening. Biological, genetic, and environmental factors influence eating disorders. Cultural influences about body image and work-related needs to keep a certain body weight contribute to eating disorders. For example, dancers have a higher incidence of eating disorders than the general population. But, men and women of all ages can have eating disorders. Here, I will discuss Anorexia Nervosa, Bulimia Nervosa, Binge Eating Disorder, Pica, and Rumination Disorder.

Anorexia Nervosa

A patient with anorexia may be easily recognized but not easily understood. It is difficult to comprehend an individual repressing a nearly undeniable instinct of hunger to the point of death. The characteristic thoughts and behaviors of anorexia nervosa patients are extreme and conflicting. They center around the sufferer's belief that they are overweight, along with an anxious desire to lose weight when they are actually underweight. Even when they lose a lot of weight and become visibly thin, they never stop believing that they are overweight and continue to be intensely preoccupied with weight loss or fear of gaining weight.

Thus, the inherently contradicting ideas of being underweight, but with a preoccupation of being overweight and trying to lose further weight, constitute anorexia. The patients are "obsessed" with weight and weight loss in the colloquial sense of obsession, meaning an intense worry and constant preoccupation, but not in terms of irrational, intrusive thoughts, like in OCD. The preoccupation and behavior may resemble the behavior of addiction, but they are not chasing a high.

Anorexia is common among teenagers and rarely found among people older than 40 or younger than 12. It is lot more common in women than in men. It is common in occupations where weight and fitness are important, like athletics, modeling, and the entertainment industry. Sometimes a stressful event or an internal or external pressure can precipitate this.

It might start as a benign or routine weight loss plan for the summer or prom, but it can cross the line when they continue their weight-loss efforts even after achieving the desired weight. At this point, once they reach the desired weight, they become less open about dieting and weight loss, as if they cross a line of logic to enter a world of unrealistic ideas about body size. Now, they might start denying their intention to lose weight, exaggerate their food intake, and avoid confrontation or discussion about their weight, despite being preoccupied with their weight all the time.

As their illness progresses, their contradictions in thoughts and behaviors become more complex. They go to extra lengths to hide their eating problems. For example, they may restrict themselves from eating anything that has fat in it but talk all the time about fatty and greasy food as if they are experts in eating fatty food. They would plan, shop, and cook an elaborate fatty meal for friends and family, but when it comes to eating, they would come up with an excuse not to eat, lie that they already ate, or take a small piece and chew for a long time, pretending to eat. They read the food labels meticulously and know all about calories, fat burning, and exercise. In any gathering, if the talk is about food, dieting, or calories, they participate with exaggerated enthusiasm and discuss in detail about the nuances of dieting and falsely brag about eating high-calorie foods out of control. On the other hand, they may become vegan or eat extremely selectively, blaming the food industry for offering unhealthy food.

At times, they may overeat and feel very guilty about it because they "slipped" from their tight regimen. A perceived or real physical discomfort from the full stomach, along with guilt, would lead them to either induce vomiting or diarrhea to compensate for their personal failure and regain "balance." Some go on an eating binge and eat a lot of food only to follow with a purging routine. The diagnostic criteria specify two types: restricting type and binge eating type, but a lot of patients overlap in their behavior.

When asked or confronted, the patients would minimize or deny that they are dieting. As they are preoccupied with the way they look, they watch themselves in the mirror for long periods of time examining every part of their body with care, looking for fat or out of shape areas, even when they are extremely thin. They prefer loose and baggy clothes that do not reveal their body, as if to deny their thinness.

Although they may be logical in other areas of their personal, professional, and social life, they are illogical and irrational when it comes to eating and body weight. They may completely deny their problem, and even deny physical symptoms, such as tiredness and actually attribute it to having too much fat in their body. Their thinking and logic become skewed towards supporting their behavior to the point where it is unclear whether they fully comprehend their contradicting thoughts.

The physical symptoms of anorexia are related to weight loss. The patients are thin, anemic, and may have tiredness and dizziness. They may have unhealthy, dry and scaly skin, hair and bone loss, and other symptoms of malnutrition, dehydration, and low blood pressure. Absence of menstrual periods used to be a sign of anorexia, but it is no longer required for a diagnosis. Some of these complications may not be reversible after they start eating. When patients die of anorexia, they die from physical complications.

Behaviorally, these patients become withdrawn and reclusive, avoiding all those who may confront them about their body weight and get very upset when confronted. They may develop emotional problems such as depression and anxiety and may exercise excessively despite failing health. The individuals with binging and purging type are prone to impulsive behaviors such as drug use or indiscriminate sex, and they may resort to self-injurious behavior.

Co-occurrence of other mental illnesses such as depression, anxiety, drug use, personality disorders, and impulse control issues is common. A high number of patients with anorexia have a history of abuse as children, including psychological, physical, and sexual abuse.

The treatment of anorexia is complex and typically involves intense psychotherapy. There are no proven medications, but medications targeting associated psychological symptoms such as depression are warranted. When the condition is acute and physically destabilizing such as in severe anorexia, they may need hospitalization and even parenteral nutrition. Cognitive behavioral therapy to help restructure the thinking of the patient as well as family-based intervention, especially in adolescents, can help patients with anorexia.

For anorexia, SSRIs such as fluoxetine, paroxetine, or citalopram are not known to help regain weight, but these are frequently used, especially when there is a component of depression or anxiety. Olanzapine, an antipsychotic with severe weight gain and sedation as side effects, seems to help anorexics regain weight. Quetiapine, an antipsychotic similar to olanzapine regarding sedation and weight gain as side effects, is also seen to be helpful for some patients. Although patients with anorexia are not psychotic, antipsychotics such as olanzapine and quetiapine seem to help them make beneficial changes in behavior and thought patterns related to impaired body image issues. Studies have shown a reduction in anxiety and depression symptoms with the use of antipsychotics in patients with anorexia.

Family Based Psychotherapy

Family-based psychotherapy, pioneered by Maudsley hospital, has been very effective in teenagers with anorexia as well as bulimia. This treatment is conducted over a year in about 20 sessions while the patient is living with their parents and siblings. The family-based approach is described in three phases; 1) weight restoration to address physical issues, 2) restoring control of eating by the patient, and 3) focusing on the normal development of the teen. In the first phase, the focus is on weight restoration and addressing physical complications of extreme weight loss. In this phase, the patient and family are observed for behavioral issues around eating.

The teen is helped to understand their conflict about weight and eating. Family members are advised to empathize with the patient's conflict and struggle but remain insistent on eating regularly and re-gaining weight. Such a combination of full understanding and sympathy as opposed to frustration and anger, without giving up on eating adequate food, seems to get them back on track to regain weight. The patient is not blamed, and the problem of eating and weight gain is externalized. Siblings and peers are educated to support the patient. The patient is expected to gain 90% of their weight and reduce anxiety and conflict about overeating before moving to the next stage.

In the second phase, more autonomy is given to the patient, and parents are involved in helping the patient regain control of eating. As the patients gain weight, the teen is given more autonomy and less supervision from the parents, but the patient is expected to continue to gain weight or maintain it. Starvation is not accepted, and patients are held accountable for eating. As the patient continues to improve and eats regularly, the focus of the treatment is moved to phase three.

In phase three, the teen comes back to the normal developmental process, which is usually interrupted in these patients. The issues of focus in this phase may extend beyond eating behavior and the behavior's impact on the patient's life.

The family-based approach may not be appropriate for grown adults living on their own. Comorbid depression, anxiety, or drug use should be addressed if present. Psychotherapy is key, and cognitive behavioral therapy seems to be effective. The treatment should focus on the central idea of the patient's body image and thought process. The treatment needs to be intense and closely monitored, with regular and frequent appointments.

The treatment of eating disorders may resemble the treatment of drug addiction and rehabilitation in some ways, although the goal in this case is for the patients to consume. Patients may resist the idea of having a disorder and the need for treatment in early stages. Quite often, patients may have a lot of physical problems by the time they come for treatment. These patients are better treated in specialized inpatient and outpatient centers.

Bulimia Nervosa and Binge Eating Disorder

Binge eating with purging behavior is known as bulimia nervosa, and without purging it is known as binge eating disorder. A binge eater consumes a very large quantity of food in a short period of time for no particular reason other than the act of bingeing. Patients with binge eating disorder are excessively worried about weight and food consumption. They try very hard to control what they eat and maintain a strict discipline about food intake. When they binge, they see themselves as a failure and feel a loss of control. Such a loss of control may happen following stress or a personal hardship. It seems that the patients are conflicted about food and eating, try to exert tight control over their eating behavior, but lose that control under stress or duress and go on a binge, as if finding a secret solace by doing something forbidden, which in turn induces guilt, leading to purging. While purging may relieve the guilt momentarily, it worsens already negative self-esteem and the feeling of failure of the self-imposed discipline. The whole process becomes a cycle and the conflict worsens. They become very secretive in their eating and purging behavior and feel disgusted with themselves.

On the one hand, it may appear that the illness is different from anorexia, but there is a lot of overlap. Besides having severe body image disturbance and conflicts about weight and dieting these disorders overlap in symptomatology. Patients with anorexia can go on binges and purges and patients with bulimia sometimes restrict food intake trying to lose weight. Some patients with bulimia may be overweight.

Bulimia is also predominantly found in young women and there is a significant co-occurrence of emotional problems like depression, anxiety, personality disorders, and drug abuse. A large number of patients have history of abuse. Social and occupational (athletes and performance artists) pressures also contribute to the illness.

The treatment of bulimia resembles that of anorexia, but SSRIs are shown to help patient with bulimia and binge eating disorder. Sometimes, the purging behavior can be very troublesome, and patients may need hospitalization or intensive supervised treatment.

Pica

Pica is an unusual eating disorder, in which the patient has some kind of craving for a non-nutritional, nonfood item for no particular reason. The patients describe the urge and need to eat the nonfood item such as chalk, clay, paint, etc., that occurs as an impulse, and they report being satisfied by or even enjoying the taste of the nonfood item they consume. They also describe an urge or craving for the specific product (be it toothpaste or false ceiling) and describe enjoying a peculiar "taste" from these materials, which is not a conventional taste sensation, but more like a metallic state. They do admit to liking the taste and being satisfied after eating the tasteless material.

Pica is frequently found in babies, children (some with nutritional deficiencies, especially iron deficiency), the developmentally disabled (mental retardation), pregnant women, and people with iron-deficiency anemia. Technically, pregnancy, iron-deficiency anemia, and developmental disability such as autism are exclusionary for a DSM diagnosis of pica, but there is no scientific evidence that differentiates pica in these situations to pica that occurs with no associated cause. It is the convention of DSM to exclude a diagnosis if it is associated with a medical condition. This convention may or may not be meaningful in some cases, but the origin is from the thinking of organic vs. nonorganic causes of psychiatric symptoms (e.g. hallucinations from epilepsy vs. psychosis).

Pica can happen in otherwise healthy people and is frequently seen among people in chemotherapy or those with chronic medical illnesses. It lacks of a clear psychological (emotional or behavioral) explanation. Pica may be related to the behavior of animals known as "salt lick" or "mineral lick," where animals seek out and lick salt or mineral deposits to consume essential minerals or salt. There is no specific treatment, and when the underlying cause, such as iron deficiency, is treated, patients improve. The patients are embarrassed and hide the behavior. Reassurance and education about safety in eating is helpful.

Patients may develop toxicity, bowel problems, or dental problems from this unusual habit. Treatment varies depending upon the individual; children and developmentally disabled individuals may benefit with restraints and reinforcing behavioral interventions, while others may benefit from education and treatment of underlying causes.

Rumination Disorder

Rumination disorder is characterized by the regurgitation, not vomiting, of food materials as a habit. Patients may chew and swallow back or spit the food. The behavior seems to be more of a habit, which is at least partly under the individual's control, and does not seem to be associated with any body image disturbance or any specific purpose (nutritional or emotional) other than the act itself. The treatment approach must be essentially behavioral, more or less like helping someone who chews fingernails. The patients need to take stock of their behavior, monitor their behavior, and inhibit and distract themselves to avoid the rumination.

Chapter 10

Alcoholism and Substance Use Disorders

"I am amazed at the varied responses I see when we use morphine to patients having a heart attack. Most patients just feel less pain. But, every now and then, a patient will say "What did you just give me doc? I feel really good." And I wonder whether these are the kind of patients at risk for addiction."

Benoy J. Zachariah
Interventional Cardiologist, Boston

To think about it, addiction is difficult to understand. At one end, so many lose their lives to addiction, while a lot of people don't even want to try a drug once or curious about the high. The very idea of a high itself evokes strong and extremely variable responses, from an intense desire with a pleasant and positive expectation to a loathsome, fearful aversion. The majority of people are very afraid of becoming addicted and refuse to take anything with an addiction potential, even when necessary. Even among users, only a small minority become problem users. Something like 80% of alcohol produced is consumed by just 2% of people who drink and, only about 38% of the population drink. Yet, addiction is one of the major psychosocial problems in any society. The use and acceptance of alcohol and drugs vary across cultures and even within a society over time. In the United States, the cultural attitude towards alcohol has significantly changed since the Prohibition era of the 1920s.

Today, attitudes created by the War on Drugs in the '80s are seemingly being rewritten as cannabis gains legalization state by state. Addiction is not a problem of the modern society, and it has been reported since ancient times. However, the legal ramifications and medical understanding of these addictive behaviors are modern and evolving. In addition, the modern "advances" in production, and refinement of the addictive substances (Heroin, cocaine from coca leaves and high potency cannabis) and the economics of the drug industry lead to more incidences of addiction.

Psychologically, addiction is defined as the preoccupation about the next fix. A heroin user may constantly and compulsively seek the drug and a binge drinker may patiently wait and plan for the drinking session over the weekend. Without the drug, for these people, life is a painful void but with the drug life becomes an unmanageable ordeal of agony and despair. These individuals live their lives in constant misery and struggle, at times, even years after they quit. What happens in the brains of those addicted is not fully understood. The drugs of abuse, in general, produce a high by activating the reward system in the brain. This phenomenon becomes a strong motivator for the addict to come back to the drug again and again, and such a need may become irreversible, meaning the patient is impaired to a point that they cannot live without the drug.

The essential feature of addiction or the more preferable term of substance use disorder is that the individual continues to use a substance in spite of experiencing significant problems from the use. The problems resulting from the addiction can be purely physical or physiological such as liver damage, or behavioral, social or psychological. But, quite often, long before such damage occurs, or long before a patient can be identified as having a substance use disorder, individuals themselves and families and friends notice a problematic drinking (or drug use). Clinically this is referred to as pathological pattern of substance use, implying that the patient has crossed the line of recreational use of drugs to a problematic use.

The DSM V criteria of substance use disorders has a comprehensive approach encompassing the social, psychological and physiological aspects of substance use with 11 different criteria. Of these 11, only two are required to make a diagnosis of substance use disorder, emphasizing the diversity in psychopathology. They are grouped under loss of control, social problems, dangerous or risky use and physiological or pharmacological impact of the drug.

Under loss of control, there are four criteria including (1) excessive or prolonged consumption, (2) awareness of such excessive use and a desire or attempts to cut down, (3) spending a lot of time around the substance including obtaining, using, and recovering from the effect and (4) craving.

Craving can be related to the aforementioned preoccupation. Craving is an intense desire and need for the drug and its effect, which becomes more of a distress if not satisfied, although the craving often passes in due time. Craving can occur randomly or when someone is reminded of the drug use, and it especially gets worse around the social or situational cues of the drug of use (for example, coffee or a heavy meal that makes one crave for cigarettes) indicating behavioral and associative learning aspect of the drug use. Craving may involve both psychological and physical dependence. Craving can become so intense that it consumes the person's time entirely to a point that he or she cannot think of anything else. Craving can persist even years after quitting. Frequent and intense cravings are good predictors of relapse, and so craving is a major issue to deal with in substance abuse treatment, recovery and relapse prevention.

The main criteria under social impairment is a (5) failure to fulfill one's duties such as work, schoolwork or family related responsibilities, (6) an impairment in interpersonal relationship and (7) compromise in personal, social and recreational activities that the individual may engage in otherwise.

In the risky use group include use of the substance in unsafe situations such as driving or while at work (8) and continued use of alcohol or a drug despite such use is harmful to the body (9). There are patients who develop cirrhosis from alcohol use, get a new liver transplanted and develop cirrhosis again by continued drinking.

Tolerance (10) and withdrawal (11) are the two criteria in the physiological or pharmacological group.

Tolerance

Tolerance is essentially a phenomenon in which the body gets used to the drug and it needs more and more for the same desired effect, or the same amount produces less of an effect. Not all drugs develop tolerance, and some drugs, notably cannabis can sometimes have something known as "reverse tolerance," meaning second use, or later use gives a better high. This is believed to happen because the first time the liver enzymes are activated which are needed to convert the cannabis into active ingredients for the brain. But this does not typically go on and on and those who consume cannabis quickly develop tolerance.

Development of tolerance may not always reflect a problem of addiction. For example, there are some patients who regularly take a prescription medication for anxiety (Lorazepam or alprazolam) or for pain (narcotic opioid painkillers) for a long period of time. These patients are most likely to be tolerant to a point that the drugs do not have any euphoric effect or high. They may or may not any have therapeutic value or effect, meaning they may or may not work for anxiety or pain. However, the patients may have become dependent on these medications meaning, if they stop, they would experience the anxiety or pain, which can be from the withdrawal. This is an interesting dilemma - which came first? Are they anxious because the original anxiety comes back? Are they anxious because they are withdrawing from the drug? Anyhow, the patients have a hard time quitting. They may be dependent, but not necessarily addicted, because they do not take it for a buzz. A low maintenance dose of these drugs, used for a long time, may not be a problem, but even in such situations, a higher than an acceptable dose (like 3 mg of lorazepam or more) may be a problem, they may be managing their dependence. These patients on such high doses are usually problematic and would certainly experience severe withdrawal. They generally do not like it if you recommend a dose reduction. Considering all these, individual patients need to be evaluated carefully.

Withdrawal

Withdrawal is a characteristic physiological syndrome that is related to the drug of intake. Withdrawal happens because an individual maintains a certain blood level of a substance for a long period, during which, the brain gets used to the externally supplied drug, and accommodates itself by reducing the internal production or changing the receptors. When the external supply is abruptly stopped, the brain may or may not revert back to original level and so, causes an artificial paucity leading to withdrawal symptoms. These symptoms vary depending on the drug.

A sudden stoppage of the (external supply of) drug can cause intense physiological distress along with craving, both of which are relieved by use of the drug or its analogue. Withdrawal from drugs like alcohol, opioids, anxiolytics and hypnotics or what sometimes referred to as "downers" because they slow down a few physiological functions of the body such as heart rate and breathing, are more easily measurable because the withdrawal causes an increase in those physiological functions as a rebound phenomenon. On the contrary, withdrawal from stimulants such as amphetamine, cocaine or nicotine may be less bothersome physiologically. The psychological withdrawal that includes intense craving and distress varies among individuals. Cannabis is a stimulant, although some users may feel that it is more sedating or slowing them down. Cannabis withdrawal with irritability, anger, anxiety, sleep problems and restlessness, is a well-documented phenomenon.

Withdrawal and tolerance are not essential to diagnose a substance use disorder. On the other hand, recreational or limited use of drugs that can harm someone (risky use) because of cultural or religious restriction, age, occupation etc, needs to be addressed in therapeutic terms.

In some ways, addiction follows the same principles of other mental illnesses such as depression and anxiety where there is a clear normal range of behavior, and in excess, the behavior is detrimental. However, it is common for everyone to feel anxiety or sadness, at times excessively, but drug use and experience of a high cannot be argued as a normal experience, thus making some feel that even recreational use of drugs and addiction is a moral issue of self-control.

Self-control, or lack of it, is a significant characteristic of people who end up being addicted to drugs. "Who is vulnerable to addiction?" is a very important question, scientifically, socially, as well as personally. Quite often we hear the term "addictive personality" denoting someone prone for addiction, which is a vague concept and is frequently misleading. Interestingly, those who worry about becoming addicted, and those who claim to have an addictive personality are actually a bit more careful in avoiding drugs of addiction, and so, are less likely to become addicted. Ironically, most of the people who are addicted to drugs or alcohol tend to deny their addiction as a problem and feel that they are not addictive and have a better control over the drug use. However, some individuals are clearly more prone to become addicted than others, and it is very common for a person who is addicted to one drug to get addicted to another.

Vulnerability to addiction has been associated with some behavioral traits such as novelty seeking, impulsivity, cue reactivity and poor self-control. There are some known factors that increase the chance of addiction in a given individual. They include genetic factors like a family history of addiction, early exposure and certainly, the environment, including availability and cultural acceptance. Comorbidity, meaning presence of another mental illness such as depression or anxiety, increases the odds of addiction. Even presence of mental illness in the family increases the odds of addiction for an individual, especially depression and anxiety within close blood relatives.

Another important psychopharmacological aspect of addiction is the route of administration and purity of the drug. For example, chewing of coca leaves that release small amounts of cocaine may build up and cause addiction more slowly than a pure or more lipophilic (a property of the drug to attach itself to fat molecule, which enhances intensity of the drug) forms of the drug like crack cocaine. Also, as opposed to chewing, smoking gives a quicker and more intense high. Similarly, intravenous heroin is a lot more rewarding (high) than swallowed opium. Addiction may not happen overnight, but it might progress rapidly when the drug is purified.

Alcoholism

Alcoholism has been a problem since modern human civilization started with organized farming about 10,000 years ago. Some believe that ancient humans discovered brewing first then invented farming techniques to supply barley and wheat for the brewing, and the rest is history. See, necessity is the mother of invention! But, considering the fact that humans are a million-year-old species it is surprising to know that he discovered beer only 10,000 years ago. Although brewing alcohol as a practice started in the "modern" society, the use of mind-altering drugs that are available in nature like mushrooms, cannabis and alkaloids have been documented since before the onset of civilization. But, the industrialization or modification of the naturally occurring substances to give a quicker and easily accessible high is certainly a modern problem.

WHO reports in 2014 that 38.3% humans consume alcohol, and on average, they consume 17 liters of alcohol per year. In 2012, it was estimated that 3.3 million people died from drinking excessively around the world, and 7.6% of deaths among men and 4% of deaths among women are attributed to alcohol. In the USA, the alcohol industry was estimated to be worth about $233 billion, but ironically, the cost of alcoholism related expense is estimated to be $244 billion (2010, from CDC). Alcoholism is certainly a major problem for the society besides being a problem for the individual and the family. People still grapple with the idea of alcoholism being a disease. This is partly because of the illness being a behavioral problem, and at times is seen as a weakness of the will power (impulse control) and so, a moral issue rather than a medical issue. Alcohol use continues to increase in the developing world and will continue to raise along with prosperity, globalization, and to an extent, westernization in the rest of the world.

Problems with drinking typically starts in teen years. Early exposure and higher tolerance are related to higher incidence of alcoholism[1]. Like many mental illnesses, alcoholism and drug addiction run in the

---

[1] Some people are less tolerant to alcohol and exhibit an unpleasant flushing reaction when they drink. This is due to a genetic variation in the enzyme called acetaldehyde dehydrogenase. Alcohol is metabolized in stages. First, it is converted into acetaldehyde by an enzyme called alcohol dehydrogenase or ADH. Acetaldehyde is a harmful byproduct, but it is short lived because it is further metabolized quickly into acetate by another enzyme called acetaldehyde dehydrogenase. Acetate is further metabolized into carbon dioxide and water. While this happens in everyone, those with this genetic variation in acetaldehyde dehydrogenase do not metabolize acetaldehyde effectively. Among these, acetaldehyde can accumulate up to 40 to 100 times normal level which causes the flushing reaction. Such flushing reaction is common among Asians with almost all Japanese, a majority of Koreans and Chinese and smaller proportion of Indians and Thai affected. Naturally this protects some from drinking heavily. Those who have flushing, and drink heavily have higher chance of cancer because acetaldehyde is carcinogenic.

families and genetic influence of alcoholism and drug addiction is estimated to be about 40 to 60%. The odds of susceptibility to addiction increase with the number of individuals affected in the family, the genetic proximity (or closer the relationship like parents and identical twins), as well as the severity of the addiction. Alcoholism is also common among families with high incidence of depression and anxiety thus illustrating a genetic overlap of these disorders.

Comorbidity is high among individuals with alcohol use disorder and drug use. Patients with a mental illness have higher incidence of alcoholism and patients suffering from addiction have higher incidence of mental illnesses. In addition, anxiety, depression, other addictions or impulse control problems such as gambling are more common among patients with alcoholism. These illnesses quite often precede the alcohol use supporting the idea of self-medication, but alcoholism also is also known to lead people for depression and anxiety disorders.

Alcoholism can lead to psychosis and dementia by its direct toxic effect on the brain. Heavy drinkers can have memory problems known as Korsakoff syndrome (actually due to vitamin B1 deficiency). They can develop gastritis, dyspepsia, liver problems leading to cirrhosis. Many people die from the effects of cirrhosis, esophageal varices, and ascites. Women in general are more susceptible to the effect of alcohol because of their low body weight, higher fat ratio, lower water content and lower metabolism in the stomach.

As discussed earlier, a diagnosis of alcohol use disorder is made if 2 of the 11 criteria are met (consuming larger amounts or for longer periods than intended, desire and effort to cut down, great deal of time spent on obtaining, drinking and recovering, failing to meet responsibility, using while having social or interpersonal problems, giving up occupational or recreational roles, using when physically dangerous, using with physical or psychological problems, craving, tolerance and withdrawal). Mild if the person meets 2 or 3, moderate with 4 or 5 and severe with 6 and above.

A lot of people including moderate drinkers suffer through the dilemma of drinking too much or being annoyed by friends and family. Some of them, including moderate or heavy drinkers stop drinking for some reason such as crisis in life, religious obligation like lent, etc., and restart on a limited basis with controlled drinking. Some heavy drinkers stop after one DUI (Driving Under Influence) charge and others learn to control. It is only a small minority that cannot control their drinking and lose everything in their lives. At times, someone like this may influence the perception about alcohol and drug addiction for the entire society. While it can be argued that it is the price society pays for the pleasure it can also be argued that the price is too much. This is a frequent sociological debate in which the families and friends of alcoholics may support the idea of a total ban of alcohol - which may never happen.

General Principles of Treatment for Substance Use and Alcoholism

Acute Withdrawal

Acute withdrawal is treated physiologically. In general, an analogue to the drug of use is given at tapering doses to ease the withdrawal symptoms until they disappear. Technically this is a controlled weaning. The physiological effects of withdrawal might disappear or reduce to a manageable level in 2 or 3 days or in about a week but the psychological effects like craving may last a long time. Benzodiazepines are used for alcohol withdrawal as well as withdrawal from other "downers" including benzodiazepine addiction. Many addictionologists use phenobarbital for benzodiazepine withdrawal, but this may not be necessary under controlled conditions like inpatient detoxification. Using alcohol withdrawal scale such as CIWA scale helps in the use of benzodiazepines. Other medications like gabapentin and anti-epileptics such as valproic acid are used on occasions. Librium is used traditionally but, in my opinion, there is no advantage to use chlordiazepoxide (Librium) over any other benzodiazepines such as lorazepam or diazepam. At times oxazepam is used for patients who have liver problems, such as cirrhosis because oxazepam skips one step of liver metabolism.

Alcohol withdrawal and withdrawal from other "downers" like benzodiazepines can cause seizures. In addition to the seizures, delirium tremens[2] is a serious withdrawal condition and it can lead to death. Delirium can also occur in other withdrawal like opiates. Chances of delirium increase with heavier drinking or drug use, older age, and other complications like infection or poor nutrition.

Delirium is a mental confusion in which patients are disoriented to time, place and person. Common symptoms of delirium are inattention, disorientation, confusion, hallucinations - predominantly visual, sleeplessness, agitation, seizures, and autonomic symptoms such as increase in blood pressure, pulse, fever etc. These symptoms have a typical waxing and waning feature with typical worsening in the evenings and nights, referred to as sun-downing. Tactile hallucinations or false feelings of things on or under the skin like bugs crawling can occur

---

2 "Delirium Tremens" is an ironically named beer by an old Belgian brewery even regarded as one of the best in the world. While it is a nice beer, I kind of cringe when I see it as it feels like a cruel joke. They also brew another beer called La Guillotine (I never knew Guillotine is feminine - La in French is feminine and Le is masculine).

frequently and are referred to "formication" (The word formication comes from Latin "formicare" meaning crawling ants). A popular form of tactile hallucination is known as "cocaine bugs" which were noted in chronic cocaine users. It can occur in any stimulant use or drug withdrawal. The treatment is similar to the treatment of withdrawal with benzodiazepines of choice[3].

Long term treatment of alcoholism and drug addiction

The long-term treatment after taking care of the withdrawal focuses on rehabilitation, maintenance of sobriety, relapse prevention and treatment of comorbid conditions. The approach of treatment in alcoholism as well as drug addiction is complex and involves a variety of approaches including medications and psychosocial interventions.

Medications

Disulfiram is an interesting medication because it does not treat any condition but acts as a deterrent by causing a reaction similar to hangover. Disulfiram blocks the breakdown of acetaldehyde produced during alcohol metabolism and toxic acetaldehyde accumulates quickly causing the typical reaction. The patients would feel severe and unpleasant flushing, headache, nausea, vomiting, breathing difficulty, sweating, palpitation, thirst, and general discomfort. Some may faint or get confused. Sometimes, patients are given disulfiram and then alcohol to let them go through this reaction to condition them to fear alcohol. This works by helping the patient or by scaring the patient from drinking.

Naltrexone is an opioid antagonist, meaning it blocks opioid receptors in the brain, but it is unclear how this works to reduce the craving of alcohol or opiates. It is believed that it works on the reward system of the brain to reduce craving. It is an antagonist as opposed to methadone and buprenorphine, which are agonists or act similar to opioids and so replace or compensate the effects of opioids and so keeps the patient from craving for them.

Acamprosate is another drug possibly working through GABA receptors that reduces craving for alcohol dependent individuals. Topiramate is an anti-seizure medication that works on GABA receptors also has been shown to reduce craving or need for alcohol. These drugs should be combined with other forms of psychosocial treatment including counseling and support.

Of the supportive treatments, the most popular and well proven method is Alcoholics Anonymous (AA). AA was started in 1935 in Ak-

[3] I once walked in to consult on a patient with polytrauma and alcohol withdrawal in a major hospital. As I was talking to the patient, a nurse walked in with two chilled cans of Budweiser beer. To avoid complications of withdrawal, the trauma surgeon routinely prescribes two cans of beer q 6 hours. Smart thinking, I thought.

ron, Ohio by Bill Wilson and Dr. Bob Smith. It is a support group where someone who is "recovering" helps others. The AA believes in recovery by a spiritual awakening. Although initially formed with Protestant beliefs, it has morphed into a non-religious, non-denominational support group that still emphasizes spirituality. Patients attend regular meetings and find a sponsor who can help one on one. The members are expected to have full commitment and the main idea behind the success of AA is that a recovering alcoholic is able to openly discuss their drinking habits and recovery to another fellow alcoholic thus helping him stop drinking. It is sometimes called as a 12-step program as it follows 12 steps starting with an admission of powerlessness over alcohol, needing a Higher Power to help them, turning self to God, identifying shortcomings, make amends with people wronged and reach a spiritual awakening. Although spiritual and religious, AA involves discipline and support, which help many individuals.

Cannabis

Cannabis is a plant that is indigenous to the Indian subcontinent where it grows wildly, thus the street name "weed." The active ingredient of cannabis is $\Delta 9$ Tetrahydrocannabinol, or THC, which causes the desired euphoric effect. Along with the euphoria, cannabis exaggerates sensory perception, making sounds and images appear more vivid, thus making it ubiquitous in music concerts. It impairs time perception, causes dry mouth, redness of eyes and makes one hungry. It is a vasodilator, and so, believed to help in maintaining erection. In the 60s, some believed cannabis to be a good aphrodisiac because of the combined effect of erection and enhanced perception. Cannabis impairs attention, judgment, cognition, and motor skills, at times even after the intoxication subsides, thus severely disturbing productivity. Although many artists claim to have good inspiration while intoxicated, they report a significant reduction in productivity while under the influence, implying the use of cannabis to be a recreational tool rather than a performance enhancer. The idea of cannabis enhancing creativity is hotly contested, especially by those who use regularly, but well controlled studies clearly show that people who smoke cannabis perform poorly on cognitive tests. Tolerance and physical dependence are not major problems with cannabis. But chronic users report irritability, poor sleep and an increase in anxiety and depression upon withdrawal.

Cannabis is a stimulant and although people report sleeping better on cannabis, the physiological nature of the sleep is impaired under its influence. Many claim a reduction in anxiety while under the influence, but for some, cannabis can be highly anxiety provoking. Some are perturbed with the paranoia it causes. While it is possible that different people respond differently to cannabis, it is not a safe anxiolytic. Cannabis is proven to make psychosis worse and cause relapse in patients with schizophrenia, despite the claims of some feeling "relaxed and better" under its influence. Availability of cannabis increases the incidence of addiction in general although marijuana advocates may dispute the idea of gateway drug. Interestingly, it has been observed that there are fewer opioid overdose deaths in states where cannabis is legalized for medical or recreational reasons.

Cannabis and psychosis

Heavy cannabis use (as well as possibly some other drugs of abuse) in younger age (between 10 and 15 years) may precipitate or even cause psychosis and schizophrenia. I have personally seen patients who smoked marijuana for 5 years or more between ages 10 and 18 develop psychosis not different from schizophrenia, get hospitalized, experience complete remission with treatment and abstinence from cannabis. They promptly relapse when they start smoking again. It is unclear whether marijuana causes psychosis or just unravels the underlying schizophrenia[4].

Opioids

Opioids are some of the most addictive substances available. The term opiates or opioids come from the word opium which is a resin from poppy plant. Opium is an alkaloid with very intense analgesic and euphoric effects. Opium has been consumed for recreational and medicinal purposes for a long time, even pre-civilization era. It was rampant in the 1700s and 1800s[5].

Opium derivatives (opiates) and synthetic or semi-synthetic molecules that resemble opium (opioids) act on several types of opioid receptors. Of them, MU (μ) receptors are believed to be responsible for analgesia, euphoria, dependence, respiratory depression and constipation. Delta (Δ) opioid receptors also seem to be involved in analgesia and physical dependence. The Kappa (κ) receptors are believed to be responsible analgesia, depression, sedation and diuresis. There are two

---

4 Several mental illnesses are related to problems in the maturation of the brain and it is wise not to use any drugs until age 25 or at least age 18. For this reason, some psychopharmacologists are leery about using stimulants in youngsters diagnosed with ADHD, especially high doses. It is not uncommon to see teens becoming psychotic from stimulants such as methylphenidate. Usually the psychosis goes away when they stop the stimulants.

5 East India Company, which was behind the eventual British rule of the Indian subcontinent, made its money by buying opium in Calcutta and selling them in China. In the 1800s, and until the communist rule, China was grappled with opium addiction. Millions and millions of people spent their days and day's wages in the opium dens.

more types identified as Nociceptin receptor that is responsible for anxiety, depression, and appetite and Zelta (ζ) receptor is believed to have a role in growth (tissue growth), embryonic development, wound repair and cancer.

There are at least three different types of opioids that are body's own, endorphins, enkephalins and nociceptins. Endorphins are secreted during acute injuries to help ease the pain. Some claim that the runner's high, a feeling of euphoria that comes after exercise comes from a secretion of endorphins. The idea is disputed, and some believe that it may be from the endogenous cannabinoids.

Opioid addiction is one of the strongest and dangerous addictions. People lose everything from wealth to home to career to modesty to this drug. Opioid addiction and overdose deaths have become epidemic in the USA since 2010s. In 2013, more people died of prescription drug abuse than street drugs. In 2014, 1.9 million people were addicted to opioid painkillers, and about 586,000 were addicted to heroin. Drug overdose was the number one cause of accidental deaths in 2014 with 18,893 overdose deaths from prescription opioids and 10,574 overdose deaths from heroin. Prescription opioid drug dependence has reached to alarming proportions in the USA. Dentists and physicians in the US are more willing to write prescriptions for narcotics than in other countries. First ever Surgeon General's report on alcohol use finds that addiction is a bigger problem than cancer.

Opioid overdose is a medical emergency and most of the deaths in opioid addiction happens due to accidental overdose. The major problem is respiratory suppression and should be handled by providing an adequate airway or ventilation until naloxone (not naltrexone), an opioid antagonist that reverses the overdose effects immediately is available. Naltrexone is also an opioid antagonist (although both naloxone and naltrexone have metabolites that are opioid agonists) but it has a long half-life and it is used as a daily pill for the maintenance treatment. It also comes as a long acting injection. Naltrexone is proven to control cravings and is used in various addictions and even for weight loss. It is not effective for the immediate use for overdose.

Opioid withdrawal is a painful condition, popularly known as cold turkey[6]. The patients feel excessive pain, chills and hot flashes,

---

6 The temperature's rising - The fever is high
Can't see no future - Can't see no sky - My feet are so heavy - And so is my head
I wish I was a baby - I wish I was dead -Cold turkey has got me on the run
Cold turkey has got me on the run - My body is aching
Goose pimple bone - I can't see nobody
Leave me alone My eyes are wide open
I can't go to sleep - One thing I'm sure of

sweating, diarrhea, nausea, vomiting, watering of the eyes and nose, muscle cramps along with insomnia and anxiety. Opioid analogues like buprenorphine, methadone or codeine immediately relieve these symptoms. Clonidine (0.1 mg to 0.6 mg a day based on the withdrawal symptoms), an alpha-adrenergic agonist relieves most of the withdrawal symptoms. Symptomatic treatment is required with NSAIDs for pain, antidiarrheal medications and proper hydration. These withdrawal symptoms improve in 2-3 days. The long-term treatment of opioid addiction follows the same principles of alcoholism with NA meeting and support.

The long-term treatment with opioid analogues such as methadone or buprenorphine to control the craving and dependence is controversial, as the idea behind using these drugs is a "replacement" or substitution. These drugs do have an addiction potential, and so are dispensed under supervision. As the patients continue to be dependent on these and are just substituting these for the street drugs, it is seen as a society sponsored addiction or dependence. Patients can be weaned off from these in the short or long run, and some remain sober successfully. Methadone is administered in specialized clinics and is not dispensed with the patient due to its addiction potential. Buprenorphine is available in combination with naloxone, which is administered sublingually. Naloxone is deactivated orally, and so they get the agonist effect from the buprenorphine but not the antagonist effect of naloxone. This is made to prevent patients from injecting the drug, as the naloxone would counteract buprenorphine. These can be used in withdrawal and long term.

Other drugs of abuse
1. Benzodiazepines
2. Barbiturates
3. Cocaine
4. Amphetamine like stimulants
   a. MDMA
   b. Khat
   c. Bath salt
5. Hallucinogens
   a. LSD
   b. Mushrooms

I'm in at the deep freeze - Cold turkey has got me on the run (repeat)
Thirty-six hours - Rolling in pain - Praying to someone - Free me again I'll be a good boy
Please make me well - I promise you anything
Out of this hell Cold turkey has got me on the run (repeat)
Songwriters: John Lennon Cold Turkey lyrics © Sony/ATV Songs LLC

6. GHB
7. Anabolic steroids.
8. Synthetic Marijuana

Benzodiazepines

Benzodiazepines are prescription medications commonly used for anxiety. They are God-sent pills that help a lot of people as safe sedatives, but they can also be highly addictive. They help in a variety of situations including, anxiety, insomnia, agitation, pre-anesthesia, alcohol withdrawal and seizures. They are some of the most commonly used and abused prescription drugs. It is a synthetic compound that acts on GABA (Gamma Aminobutyric Acid) receptors to cause the desired sedation or sleep. The use and misuse of benzodiazepines is discussed elsewhere. It is important to remember that any benzodiazepine can be safely used for short term. A regular use beyond a few weeks should be considered as an issue of dependence although many patients with anxiety or seizures may need this for years or for the rest of their lives. In such cases it is important that they do not increase the dosage. A dose escalation - meaning an increase in the dose to reach the same effect (of sedation or sleep for example) is a sign of dependence.

Barbiturates

Barbiturates are CNS depressants, more or less like benzodiazepines which essentially replaced barbiturates for all its therapeutic uses. Barbiturates have anxiolytic, sedative and hypnotic properties. In the past, they were heavily used for anxiety and sleep, but due to its addiction potential, and overdose risk it is not prescribed as much. It is still used in epilepsy, general anesthesia and occasionally in the treatment of benzodiazepine withdrawal[7].

Cocaine

Cocaine is the white powder seen in Hollywood movies, where someone separates it with a razor blade on a hand mirror to make a "line" and snort it (just in case if you did not know). It is a powerful stimulant, and the white powder is a water-soluble hydrochloride salt that can be snorted or injected. When this salt is treated with baking soda or ammonia, it forms a freebase called crack cocaine. Crack cocaine is smoked in a pipe and the name crack comes from the crackling noise it makes when smoked. It is highly addictive as the purified form.

Coca leaves have been chewed for millennia in south and central America. After cocaine was extracted in 1859, it was thought to be an ex-

---

[7] Barbiturates were popular drugs of addiction in the '70s and is a main feature of the famous book and movie "Valley of the Dolls" in which the word doll is indirectly referred to barbiturates like Seconal that was known in the streets as dolls.

cellent medicine and was used in tonics, elixirs and tinctures. Coca cola had cocaine in its early preparation and even today, a flavoring agent extracted from coca leaves (without the cocaine) is used in coca cola. Coca leaves were used by and distributed for physical laborers in South America[8]. Again, the modern science has helped us to extract and refine the best "stuff" out of the relatively less dangerous naturally occurring drug to highly effective and highly addictive drug.

Cocaine is very high in addiction potential. Cocaine increases dopamine levels in the brain reward circuitry. Dopamine is a neurochemical that brings forth the good feeling of winning, be it scoring a goal, video games or just rewarding yourself. Cocaine increases dopamine to a very high-level causing euphoria, but chronic use may harm this reward circuitry.

Cocaine is very short acting and the high when snorted lasts for about 30 to 60 minutes and 15 to 30 minutes when smoked. The high is described as an immediate and intense happiness or euphoria, with high energy and alertness. It can cause heightened sensitivity to sensory stimuli, paranoia or psychosis. The withdrawal and physical dependence are subtle with a strong psychological component but can still cause strong addiction.

Amphetamine Type Stimulants

Amphetamine and similar synthetic molecules such as methamphetamine (crystal meth), dextroamphetamine (Adderall), Lisdexamfetamine (Vyvanse), methylphenidate (Ritalin), MDMA (Ecstasy) and other synthetic drugs are all stimulants that work more or less in the same manner. They all have similar effects and side effects, varying in potency. A lot of people do not realize that Adderall and Crystal Meth are kind of cousins like oxycontin and heroin. All these stimulants are moderately addictive and may cause agitation, paranoia and psychosis at higher doses. Prescription stimulants, like prescription narcotics are used in excess in the United States but get less attention than the opioids because they are a bit less addictive and less lethal[9].

These stimulants generally increase dopamine, norepinephrine and serotonin in the reward system of the brain causing euphoria or the high. They enhance focus, alertness, and energy and suppress appetite. They increase sensory perception and sex drive. Some of them increase empathy (MDMA) or feeling of closeness with others. At higher doses,

---

[8] Henri Charrière AKA Papillon describes how coca leaves were useful for him to trek miles without getting tired or sleeping less.

[9] The issue of ADHD and stimulant use is controversial because of the addiction and psychosis. Some believe ADHD is not a disease and use of stimulants is akin to performance enhancement.

stimulants can cause paranoia and psychosis. Amphetamines and stimulants improve attention and cognition. Some people even believe that amphetamine like stimulants should be legally allowed as performance enhancers - available with or without prescription more or less like caffeine. But they all have severe addiction potential, and harmful effects on the brain and body.

MDMA (Ecstasy)

MDMA (MethyleneDioxyMethAmphetamine) is known as Ecstasy and is a popular among teens who go to clubs with loud dance music. In addition to the euphoria, MDMA enhances perception and the feelings of togetherness or empathy, which is rather unique. Such an effect has made some to believe that this can be a good thing for the world![10] MDMA is not as highly addictive as Heroin or alcohol but it is not safe. MDMA is taken as a pill and the high that starts after 30-40 minutes lasts for about 3-6 hours. Overdose (8 times the desired dose) can be fatal. A combination of high energy, increased heart rate, increase in core body temperature and dehydration can lead to death.

Khat

Khat is a very popular stimulant used in The Arabian Peninsula and the Horn of Africa. It is chewed as a fresh plant because when the leaves dry the active ingredient, an alkaloid known as cathinone decomposes into a milder form known as cathine. Cathinone is similar to amphetamine and its effect is also described to be similar with an increase in alertness, concentration and euphoria. At a higher dose or with longer use, this is known to precipitate or cause psychosis. Some users claim that this is more or less like caffeine, but it is clearly a stronger stimulant with numerous side effects, and it is not as safe as caffeine. It is legal in some Arabic and African countries.

Bath Salts

These are synthetic molecules that are similar to the Khat described above. They are also stimulants not unlike the above, but they are mostly known for the popularity or notoriety they achieved because some became psychotic and violent. It is important to remember that any of these stimulants can lead someone to psychosis and bizarre or violent behavior.

---

10 The combination apparently fuels the teens in a crowded dance floor, making them sway together with music, often with a glow stick and a silly smile on their face. There is a "rave" subculture around the drug, similar to the LSD fueled youth of the 70s, who imagined peace, love and harmony on earth. The rave subculture uses the mantra PLUR that stands for Peace, Love, Unity and Respect. Interestingly, most of the hippies of every generation sooner or later end up as suburban moms and dads driving their kids to soccer games, but no one talks about the high of the simple married life.

Hallucinogens

Hallucinogens are mind altering substances that alter the perception of things around, and sometimes, things that are not around. These drugs induce a high along with unusual experiences, that are, in general, pleasant and euphoric. Some natural hallucinogens have been used in various cultures over the years to induce a spiritual experience. Sometimes profound, these spiritual experiences can have a strong impact on people. Much has been written by the drug users about how these hallucinogens, particularly LSD, induce a transformation of consciousness, expansion of the self, multidimensional thinking, experiences in different planes of reality, mystical awakening of the inner spirits, and so on and so forth. These may sound rather crazy and unreal for non-users, but one can imagine what these drugs make one feel.

Other Drugs

1. Ayahuasca: Ayahuasca is a concoction used by some Amazonian indigenous people for religious sacrament and religious experience. It contains dimethyltryptamine (DMT), which is a serotonin analogue. DMT is synthesized in labs and sold in the streets as Dimitri.

2. LSD: LSD is the most celebrated drug of all hallucinogens or psychedelics. LSD fueled counterculture or drug subculture of the 1970s along with the free spirits and hippie movements around the time of Vietnam war, producing some of the most popular music, art and pop culture that may have changed the history of mankind and may have contributed to the war on drugs of the 1980s. The psychedelic effects of LSD are attributed to its actions on dopamine and serotonin receptors. The effects of LSD are essentially based upon the individual and his or her unique experiences. But in general, people claim that the sensory perception is significantly altered or enhanced, with an exaggerated sense of reality and a sense of altered time perception.

3. Peyote: Peyote is a small spineless cactus containing mescaline, found in Mexico and southern Texas. It has been used for more than 5000 years by the indigenous people in Mexico for spiritual reasons.

4. Psilocybin: Psilocybin is the main ingredient in magic mushrooms, often touted as the drug that induces spirituality or makes one experience God.

5. Dextromethorphan is a common ingredient in cough medicine that is abused at higher than recommended doses to induce "out of body experience."

6. Ketamine: Ketamine is an anesthetic used in humans and animals. This became popular among club goers in Europe for some time. The drug is diverted from surgical and veterinary centers or drug

wholesalers to the streets. This causes dissociation, and some describe a near death experience. Ketamine is an NMDA antagonist. Ketamine is becoming popular as an antidepressant with immediate antidepressant effects.

7. Phencyclidine (PCP or Angel Dust): PCP is also an NMDA receptor antagonist that causes dissociations and hallucinations. It attained notoriety for the psychosis and violent behavior it sometimes leads to. At some point, PCP was a major problem in America and attained notoriety as a date rape drug.

8. Salvia Divinorum is a plant derivative used by Shamans in Mexico. This is a different kind of hallucinogen, acting on kappa opioid receptors. Salvia is not an alkaloid like LSD, and it does not work on the serotonin receptors. Salvia is highly potent and has psychedelic effect at less than 200 micrograms. Salvia does have a strong agonist effect of the dopamine D2 receptors.

9. Other drugs: GHB is a neurotransmitter that is closely related to GABA and acts on the GABA receptor. It is occasionally used in anesthesia and in Narcolepsy. This also has the notoriety as a date rape drug.

Synthetic Marijuana

John W Huffman, a professor at Clemson University conducted research on cannabis for medical purposes, and over time, synthesized various cannabis like molecules and published them. These publications were used to manufacture some of these compounds and are sold as synthetic marijuana. Some of these compounds such as JWH-018 are a lot more potent and so, are more dangerous than cannabis. The effects are similar to cannabis.

Anabolic Steroids

These are the "steroids" that are used by athletes and bodybuilders. These are illegal in competitive sport. There is evidence that some men obsessively exercise and excessively use anabolic steroids to a point of addiction or abuse. But, unlike other drugs of abuse, these may not cause euphoria. These improve and enhance performance, help in appearance, and, so self-esteem. These are not safe drugs and when used repeatedly, they can cause serious side effects including strokes, heart attacks, impotence and low libido.

Chapter 11

Personality Disorders

Of the many things the human brain does, the computational complexity it employs in an interpersonal interaction is astounding. Social behavior is not unique to humans, and animals do exhibit a variety social and interpersonal behaviors that help in their survival or reproduction. Packs of wolves or schools of fish are good examples. Termites and ants work together to build and protect their nests. Courting behaviors and mating rituals of some animals are fascinating. However, human social behavior and interpersonal interactions are infinitesimally complex, varied, multilayered, and nuanced, yet safe and productive, at least most of the times.

Imagine how you interact differently in a single day between family, friends, colleagues, bosses, subordinates, strangers you do not know, and strangers you just met. Our brain is capable of understanding each situation, context, and person and choose the appropriate language, attitude and demeanor. For example, we all recognize that we can get away with a strong display of discontent with our family members but not office colleagues. Quite often, even in the same situation we may behave completely differently, depending upon the person we are dealing with. For example, we may go to the same coffee shop every day but interact differently depending upon the person in the counter, their personalities or current mood. Our behaviors in those situations are influenced by our personality, as well the personality of the other person. What if such a capacity is impaired to a point it becomes harmful?

If depression is a disease of the emotional brain, and schizophrenia is a disease of the thinking part of the brain, personality disorders are diseases of the interpersonal interaction (and self-identity) aspect of the brain. A personality is defined as the "predictable pattern of interpersonal interaction" and personality disorders can be defined as "pathological patterns of interpersonal behavior."

We all know, understand, and are aware of people's personalities, certainly those who are close to us, but also people whom we just met. Good or bad, we all quickly judge someone's personality within a minute or two and adjust our behavior accordingly. We could trust, mistrust, feel attracted or repulsed for people even after a short interaction. Such a judgment depends on our personality, as well as the other person's personality, or what we choose to present or project at that point. Remember, how we behave or choose to behave is dependent upon how we see ourselves and how we want to be seen by others. Personality encompasses our own idea of self or self-identity and its complex interaction with other personalities.

These interactions form the basis of how we perceive and react to different people. Even among close friends or family, we differentiate one from another depending upon such interactions. We choose to borrow money from only a few or avoid asking certain people for favors, all depending upon their personalities. Such an expectation and mental framework is established by historical evidence in similar situations. We would have avoided people who rubbed us in the wrong manner in the past and become closer to some whose behavior had been more accommodating. The personalities and interpersonal behavior may not always be characterized as good or bad or productive or nonproductive. Someone who is manipulative may advance in their career, and so is considered productive and successful, but at the same time, not likable. Similarly, someone who is blunt and honest may have a lot more enemies even though one cannot complain about them being honest. While personality differences add diversity to society and enrich our lives, personality disorders are harmful, not only to those who have such a disorder but those who come across them.

There are several classifications of personality disorders, and the DSM classification, which includes ten disorders divided in three clusters (A, B and C), is straightforward and easy to understand.

Cluster A includes odd or eccentric personality disorders where the underlying theme is a lack of or a deficiency in the quality or quantity of the interpersonal interaction and so may not particularly be highly influencing others. They include; schizoid personality disorder, paranoid personality disorder and schizotypal personality disorder. These people are generally ignored or avoided by others.

Cluster B includes dramatic, emotional and erratic behaviors that typically evoke strong response from others, and so are either extremely attractive or strongly repulsive. They include; antisocial, borderline, histrionic and narcissistic personality disorders. These people usually impact and influence their acquaintances or even the greater society they are part of, most often in a detrimental manner.

The underlying theme of Cluster C personality disorders is anxiety and nervousness. People in this cluster are driven by fear or discomfort over themselves, quite often a discomfort for social or interpersonal interaction itself. They include; avoidant, dependent and obsessive-compulsive disorders. People in this cluster may or may not influence others like in cluster B, but they can be a source of discomfort or annoyance.

Personality and its disorders are generally enduring, consistent. The prevailing pattern of behaviors typically do not change over one's lifetime. Although the behavior can be modified or restricted to an extent by the environment, or external mechanisms such as punishment for criminal behavior, the core attitude, thought process and the pattern of emotional reaction usually last for lifetime. Such an enduring nature of the personality supports the idea that it is a biological trait like skin color, but we know very little about the biological aspects of personality.

There is no evidence for any medication helping change the personality or minimize the impact of the behaviors associated with personality disorders. However, people with personality disorders are almost always prescribed medications. Medications do help associated symptoms such as anxiety or depression. Sometimes, however, practitioners may use a different diagnosis that has more treatment options on purpose. For example, patients with schizotypal personality disorder may be diagnosed with schizophrenia and patients with borderline personality disorder may be diagnosed with bipolar illness. Some clinicians may sincerely believe in such diagnoses or overlap of such diagnoses. Quite often such "intentional" or "complicit" (false) diagnoses give hope and a feeling of purpose to the patient, as well as the treating clinician. Caution must be exercised in these circumstances to not give false or excessive hope and avoid unnecessary side effects.

Interestingly, clinicians used to avoid talking about or informing the patients of their personality disorders, partly because of the stigma, and possibly to avoid offering a diagnosis with no hope of treatment. But, these days, patients are often well informed of their personality disorder, and such an awareness seems to help more than hurt. It is not a bad clinical practice to inform patients with personality disorders of their diagnosis and educate them about realistic goals and purpose of medications.

It is very important to identify, diagnose and treat comorbid conditions such as anxiety, addiction, or depression in these patients. The effective treatment or management of personality disorders include long

Cluster A Personality Disorders

Schizoid Personality Disorder

Schizoid personality disorder is characterized by a significant lack of social or interpersonal interaction along with extremely limited emotional expression. Their problems may lie somewhere in between a lack of interest, a lack of capacity, and a lack of need or a disinterest in socialization. These people do not see the need to be social, and quite often, choose a job or are comfortable with a job that requires little socialization, like night watchmen. Unlike people with social phobia, they do not feel anxious or afraid of social situations; they just don't see the need for socialization, and they seem to lack the basic understanding of social norms and etiquette. They are emotionally cold, do not respond or appreciate praise or criticism, and do not understand others' mood or attitude appropriately. They may not have any friends other than first degree relatives and, left alone, they may not seek to have a sexual or romantic relationship. An interesting aspect of schizoid personality disorder is that affected individuals may not seek help partly because of a lack of impairment, questioning the idea of this being a disorder. These individuals may live a life of solitude, not bothering anyone and not distressed about it.

It may be very difficult to differentiate between schizoid personality disorder and mild autism, especially when the patients with autism do not have associated symptoms like ritualistic behavior etc. Technically, autism is diagnosed in childhood or even in infancy, but personality disorders are typically diagnosed at the age of 18. However, some with personality disorders do exhibit traits and behavior long before they are 18, and, some with mild autism might escape notice until later when social interaction becomes more demanding. One way to think about this is that the capacity for interpersonal interaction, or the capacity to empathize with others, are lacking in autism, and do not change much over time. Whereas, people with schizoid personality may start of as children who are shy or lacking interpersonal skills and get worse as they age. Again, this is a loose differentiation which I am forcing to employ.

This is one of the areas of ambiguity or overlap in psychiatry that may or may not have valid reason behind the thinking. To confuse further, at some point in the '80s, the ICD system had a diagnostic category called "simple schizophrenia," which is identical to schizoid personality disorder. In fact, some schizophrenia patients with prominent negative symptoms may look very similar to schizoid personality disorder. An important distinction is that, unlike patients with schizophrenia, patients with schizoid personality disorder do not exhibit thought disorder or cognitive deficits. Another important distinction is longitudinal history. Schizophrenia patients have a variable course of illness with acute psychosis, recovery, and a functional decline, whereas personality disorders do not vary a lot over time.

Schizotypal Personality Disorder

A person with schizotypal personality disorder exhibits similar behavior to schizoid personality disorder, in that the individual has a reduced capacity for social behavior. They also exhibit a variety of eccentric behavior and occasional perceptual disturbances. These are the people who are preoccupied with the unknown, occult, and metaphysical powers more so than the culture which they come from. They may have paranoid ideas or ideas of references, but none that amounts to a delusion. Stereotypical, metaphorical, pseudo-philosophical thinking and speech, along with odd, eccentric or peculiar behaviors make them stand out. They may have occasional, unusual perceptual experiences that do not amount to auditory or visual hallucinations. While they may end up leading an unusual lifestyle, they do not become psychotic as patients with schizophrenia, or become disabled. While this appears to be "schizophrenia lite," these patients do not go through the typical pattern or episodes of psychosis, remission, and relapse. Yet, they may have occasional psychosis. It is possible that this could be part of the schizophrenia spectrum disorder, but unless the core biological abnormalities of these illnesses are clearly understood, they cannot be differentiated from each other. Unlike schizophrenia, a treatment with antipsychotic medication is not very useful in these patients.

Paranoid Personality Disorder

Individuals with this illness essentially operate under suspicion. Their lives are formed and filled with suspicion or conspiracy. They constantly suspect - with no evidence - that others are plotting, harming, exploiting and deceiving them. They do not trust anyone, and so, do not confide in anyone. They suspect their spouses of infidelity, and question the loyalty of coworkers, and family members. They hold grudges, perceive personal attacks or threats from others for trivial, imagined, and irrelevant reasons. Most often, the bystander might dismiss them and their fears as baseless, exaggerated, and unnecessary paranoia, but the patients are tormented by their own fears and suspicions. They get in more trouble when they act on their suspicions, for example by confronting their spouses of infidelity. Again, medications don't always work, and therapy helps infrequently.

Cluster B Personality Disorders

The personalities or personality disorders in this cluster are the ones that get the most attention (pun intended) and the most interesting. They also are the ones that impact others and the society to a great extent. As the understanding of personality disorders advance, there will be a lot more attention paid to these abnormalities as public health concerns. In a society where malaria and cholera are eradicated, cancer is conquered and when the life-threatening illnesses are not a major problem, these personality disorders will be an area of focus. I think so, because these personality disorders bring so much misery, to not just the individuals suffering from them, but for their friends, relatives, coworkers and the greater society in general.

For example, imagine a new town is formed in some place and let us say there are about 200 families. Everybody knows everybody. No one worries about crime and no one locks the door - let us say. One day, something goes missing because someone stole or vandalized it. You can imagine the entire town reacting to this event by changing their behavior. Everyone is going to lock their doors, keep things safe, watch their backs, and talk about the thefts, spending a lot of time and effort because of one incident and one person. If that individual has antisocial personality disorder, he (most likely a he as it is more common in men) might continue to engage in criminal behavior that would permanently influence the reaction and behavior of the rest of the society. Although many people are capable of bad behavior, especially under certain circumstances, the society is shaped by the extreme behavior of just a few individuals.

Antisocial Personality Disorder

The essential feature of this personality disorder is a lack of remorse. They do not feel the need to follow social norms, rules, or obligations (thus the name antisocial. Quite often the word antisocial is used to refer to people who do not socialize much. The correct word for that would be asocial). They repeatedly engage in behaviors that are grounds for arrest or reprimand. They do not have any concern for others' feelings. They frequently con, cheat or trick others for their benefit, usually for immediate gratification, and when confronted, they find a way to rationalize their behavior and frequently blame others for their actions. An extreme example of such a rationalization is when a rapist blames the victim for lack of cooperation as a reason for their violence. People with ASPD have poor impulse control, and they pick fights and arguments easily, usually resorting to physical violence. They often use alcohol and drugs heavily, landing themselves in more trouble.

Antisocial personality disorder is a gruesome behavioral problem. Coming across one of them can send chills down the spine with fear, although sometimes with admiration as someone with ASPD can be charming, while cold-hearted. They instantly evoke fear, anger, frustration, helplessness and a serious sense of an altruistic desire to rid them of the society, unless you are one of them. These are the people who are serial criminals, con men, and petty thieves. While everyone who commits a crime may not have ASPD, people with ASPD do not live under expected social norms. Understandably, about half of men and one in five women in prisons would meet the criteria of ASPD. A high incidence of ASPD is found in patients who seek treatment for alcohol and substance abuse. Some, with ASPD, or features of ASPD may become successful in their lives, partly because they are ruthless and charming.

As they do not feel guilt or remorse, do not accept their misdeeds or take responsibility for their actions, they do not learn from their mistakes. As you can see, these people hurt others and the society, over and over for a long time. Numerous victims suffer through, at times with a lifelong scar, due to their misfortune of crossing paths with a psychopath. One can imagine the ripple effect of one individual with ASPD in a society. They pry on the innocent and gullible by making them do things and get them in trouble. They form quick relationships, but never maintain long term relationships, partly because their relationships are superficial and exploitative.

ICD calls this dissocial personality disorder and other words such as psychopath or sociopath are frequently used to describe individuals with this condition. Experts argue about subtle differences between these names, but for practical purposes and at the level of expertise of the intended audience of this book, the differences are not worthy of concern.

There is no clear treatment for ASPD or criminal behavior. A lot of research has been done in this condition, as this is a fascinating disorder and as there are many characters in history with ASPD who lived colorful lives. Society has a fascination about daredevil con men, who are serial seducers, and those who raise to the top quickly. Conmen are celebrated in pop culture - in movies and novels (who is going to care about a 9 to 5 guy with a wife and two kids in the suburb? How interesting is his life?). Some historic conmen and successful leaders are suspected to have ASPD.

ASPD, has strong genetic influence and biological roots. A high level of testosterone and a low level of serotonin has been found to be associated with ASPD. Some studies have found a correlation to closed head injuries affecting the frontal lobe. ASPD frequently precedes with conduct disorder in childhood. In fact, the behaviors are very similar and, by the criteria, a teen with conduct disorder would be diagnosed with ASPD on his 18th birthday. Description of the behavior and criteria for conduct disorder are essentially age related.

There is no proven treatment for ASPD or conduct disorder. Intervention may include treating comorbid conditions such as addiction and depression or anxiety. Some believe that people with ASPD may not develop depression because the characteristics of depression such as feeling sad, feeling guilty, empathy and introspection are contradictory to the core feature of ASPD.

Borderline Personality Disorder

Borderline personality disorder, or BPD, endures a lot of negative rap in clinical setting, more so than any other mental illness, not just because of what patients with BPD go through but because of what they make the rest of us go through. A single patient may demand the attention of the entire staff for the whole day. These patients may enter into others' lives like a storm and invariably sustain lasting damage. These patients evoke strong emotions, positive and negative, on others.

However, it is a mistake if we look at BPD from the point of view of others. Patients with BPD suffer as much as or possibly more than people with other illnesses. But, unfortunately, patients with BPD are despised, and looked at with disdain in clinical and social settings, eliciting a strong stigma even when the "rest of us" secretly desire them and feel attracted and drawn to them. Not very dissimilar to the behavior of patients with BPD, who like and dislike others to extremes with passion, we also are extremely attracted to or repulsed by the emotional ups and downs of BPD.

BPD is characterized by an instability in interpersonal relationship, poor self-image, chronic feelings of emptiness, dysregulations of mood and thought, impulsivity, anger and suicidal behavior.

Patients with BPD have poor control of their thoughts and emotions. Their emotional reactions are intense, extreme and quick. A small victory, which others might treat with a smile and a short-lived good feeling, may catapult them to an intense joy and celebration. Similarly, when they crash, they may feel doom, misery and grief over even a small day to day mishap. These extreme emotional reactions are particularly predominant in the interpersonal context but can occur in day to day circumstances, like the breakdown of a car.

A real or perceived feeling of rejection is a strong inducer of such negative emotion, at times to a point of despair and suicidal thoughts, or even suicide. Similarly, an appreciation or extra attention from someone would make them feel extreme joy and feelings of love and affection. Thus, these patients seem to have a fear of abandonment or rejection by others in the interpersonal settings. They see others, especially those who are emotionally close, as either all good or all bad, sometimes referred as black and white thinking, or splitting.

Splitting is commonly misunderstood and used to denote divide and conquer techniques. The word "splitting" here means the psychological mechanism of the individual who has poorly developed personalities such as BPD to look at people as either all good or all bad, as they have difficulty integrating the fact that people may have both good and bad aspects to them. Because of these extremes of interpersonal emotional interactions, they have chaotic, dramatic, intense, unstable and impulsive relationships. Poor impulse control is common among these individuals, and they may get in trouble with alcohol or drug use.

In BPD, the self-image and self-identity are disturbed and distorted. Self-image or sense of self is what we believe about ourselves in a greater social context. Self-image includes what we believe about who we are, what others think about us, and how we expect to conduct ourselves in society. Self-image is generally well established, unchangeable and enduring, although we may, at times, have uncertainties about self, leading to personal conflicts - especially as teenagers. But we all learn and understand our capacities and abilities and reconcile with our limitations to live in peace with ourselves. But, among people with BPD, such concept of self is unclear, broken or disintegrated leading to inconsistencies in the way they behave. Imagine yourself being stuck in a party where you do not belong. People with BPD feel like they are in the wrong party all the time because, not only can they have no clear idea of themselves, they also do not have a clear idea of their place in the rest of the society.

Individuals with BPD complain of emptiness or a void in their lives which, quite often, is misidentified as depression by the patients, as well as clinicians. They also report tension, which at times, is perceived as anxiety. An intense feeling of tension or sadness is frequently associated with self-harming behavior, like cutting the wrist. While suicide and suicidality are common in patients with BPD (6 to 10% of individuals with BPD commit suicide), most of the time, patients who cut themselves do not have a real intention to end their lives. They claim that the physical pain from a cut in the wrist relieves such tension. However, patients do report a suicidal impulse, albeit a momentary one, during

Personality Disorders

their self-injurious acts. With a variety of symptoms and behaviors that are extreme in nature, these patients use health resources disproportionately, further perpetuating the stigma.

The treatment of BPD has seen some advances recently. Dialectical Behavioral Therapy (DBT) based on Cognitive Behavioral Therapy (CBT) seems to help these patients as well as the new Mindfulness Therapy. In DBT, the therapist, helps the patient identify maladaptive thoughts, beliefs, emotions, and emotional reactions and helps them to normalize these based on facts. For example, it helps to work with the patient to see the pattern of catastrophization or idealization about things and people. They are helped to understand that, people (including themselves) cannot be all bad or all good but they are a mix of good and bad. This can be supported with group therapy, support, education and regular cognitive restructuring exercises and role plays. Groups are effective because it is easier for people to see the mis-perceptions in others than themselves, and patients feel very supported by someone else who also is having similar problems.

Mindfulness therapy or Mindfulness Based Cognitive Therapy (MBCT) is also somewhat similar, in which the patients are trained to watch (be cognizant of) their mood and thought constantly. Unrealistic negative thoughts and assumptions are identified as automatic thoughts or automatic reactions. These are maladaptive cognitive mechanisms that perpetuate negative and destructive thought and emotion. For example, a person with depression may see and react to things in live in a negative way, and even a small setback or a disappointment seem exaggerated and overwhelming[1]. Patients are helped to avoid these automatic and maladaptive reactions. Mindfulness meditation and stress reduction techniques have been gaining in popularity. As one can see, such an approach could have significant efficacy on the dysregulation of mood and thought of the patients with borderline personality disorder.

Medications, ranging from SSRIs, antipsychotics, fish oil and mood stabilizers have been used in BPD. None has been proven to help, although patients at times would claim that certain medication helped them greatly – for a short period of time. It is not uncommon for patients to have the same extreme love or hate attitude towards medications. For example, they may get way too excited about a new medication to declare that it is the best medicine that they ever took (and you are the best doctor they had ever seen) for the first week or two, only to dismiss or disregard the medicine as the worst ever (as well as you). While there is no clear evidence for any medication to help BPD, an accurate diagnosis

---

1 "In every life we have some trouble. But when you worry, you make it double" - Bobby McFerrin from "Don't worry… Be happy")

and treatment of comorbid conditions such as depression or anxiety is necessary. These individuals are prone for addiction due to impulsivity, and unfortunately, many of these patients are prescribed addictive medications such as benzodiazepines and stimulants. At times, medications may do more harm than help for these patients.

Narcissistic Personality Disorder

The word narcissism comes from the Greek Mythological character Narcissus who supposedly fell in love with himself because he was so beautiful. He became so self-absorbed he could not think of anything else. It is common for people to assume Narcissus to be a female character but, Narcissistic Personality Disorder (NPD) is more common among men.

Narcissistic Personality Disorder (NPD) is characterized by an unrealistic sense of high self-worth or self-importance. They have grandiose self-image of being unique, superior, intelligent and good looking or better looking. They seek or demand admiration and appreciation from others. They genuinely feel that everyone else is inferior and believe that anything anyone else does, they can do better. Interestingly, they may not fully feel confident about themselves, and are frequently jealous of others who are accomplished. At the same time, they may accuse others of being jealous and jeopardizing their deserved success. They frequently engage in daydreaming or spend a lot of time thinking about achieving great and spectacular success. They feel entitled, arrogant, and expect obedience from others and see others as losers and followers. They frequently manipulate others to get their way, and they disregard others' feelings by failing to empathize, even when others are hurt by their actions.

There is some evidence that people with NPD or narcissistic traits are more successful than average, and actually end up as leaders or managers. NPD is found more frequently in CEOs and leaders. The pompous and arrogant demeanor, along with manipulation and constant aspiration to move up and become prominent, enables success to some extent. Considering this, there is some argument that this disorder is only a "disorder" that affects others, but not the individual afflicted with NPD. However, people with NPD quite often possess a fragile ego that gets affected when their lofty expectations are not met, leading to misery. Yet, people with NPD very rarely get empathy and sympathy from others - even from their loved ones. We might let them lead, and tolerate them from a distance, but we generally do not like to be close to them. Narcissistic traits, on the other hand, are not always disliked,

Personality Disorders

especially from a distance. A bit of narcissism in entertainers like actors or even sportsmen are frequently admired.

Histrionic Personality Disorder

The core of Histrionic Personality Disorder (HPD) is a desire to be the center of attention in a social setting, even if it is negative attention[2]. Of the dramatic personality disorders from cluster B, HPD deserves special attention as the embodiment of drama. These individuals feel uncomfortable when they are not the main attraction of an event or social gathering. A person with HPD may not play well as a bridesmaid. They particularly feel uncomfortable when someone else is paid attention, even if it is a medical attention. For example, if someone collapses in a social gathering for genuine medical reason and, if that person is tended by doctors and paramedics with a bunch of sympathetic onlookers, these people may faint, fall, or fake an illness[3]. These individuals typically present in a flamboyant, colorful, and theatrical manner, often exaggerating their feelings and emotions.

They are seductive, using their appearance and sexuality as a tool to get attention. Interestingly, others may pay attention to the comical and exaggerated presentation and play along with them in their theatrics, but they may not have the emotional involvement or connection like in borderline personality disorder. Others may feel annoyed by their theatrics. The emotional experiences of people HPD are unstable, dramatic but shallow, and disproportionate to the actual events. Often, they are inconsiderate of others' feelings, but they get hurt easily, especially when they do not get the appreciation and attention they desire.

They are highly suggestible and are easily manipulated or influenced by others. They are egocentric and self-indulgent. They think about themselves and their appearance or presentation more than some essential things in life. For example, they often put their outward ap-

---

[2] "If it is a wedding, I have to be the bride and if it is a funeral, I have to be the corpse" - a line from a Bollywood movie, as quoted by Dr. Nagesh Mukundu

[3] Years ago, I moonlighted in a jail. One night, a patient barricaded himself in his cell and threatened to kill himself as a protest. While the ingenious guards somehow broke into the cell, saved the patient, and sent him by ambulance to the hospital, another patient with personality disorder tried to hang himself. One of the experienced guards, who went on a roll call to check on all the patients, found him almost turning blue and saved him. He told me that whenever there is a commotion like this someone always tries to do something like this. His astuteness, experience and intelligence saved this patient. However, right after we put the second patient in an ambulance, I heard a thud behind me and one of the staff nurses fell on the floor with a fake faint and claimed that her diabetes is acting up. We also put her in an ambulance and sent her to the same hospital although her blood sugar, vitals and everything else was normal. Before we sent her in the ambulance, a senior nurse had the presence of mind to check with her about the possible co pay for the ambulance ride and made sure that she was aware of the price she would have to pay for the drama...

pearance ahead of basic necessities[4]. Their lives and priorities are centered around them being the center of attention and they measure their success, or self-satisfaction by the amount of attention they get (the number of "likes" they get!). As this is a transient thing, they live by the day. They have a hard time planning for the long term and delaying the gratification. They also do not measure a success unless it is advertised. Externally, these individuals appear to be prominent, and successful, leading a grand life but internally they are unhappy, dissatisfied, discontent and miserable, with a chronic feeling of inadequacy.

Cluster C Personality Disorders

Personality disorders in this cluster differ from the eccentric cluster A, and the dramatic or emotional cluster B by the pattern of interpersonal behavior driven by anxiety, nervousness and fear. These may be the people commonly referred as "anal" type[5]. These are the people who are meticulous, prompt, well organized, and well prepared, but still worry that they are not ready. You may have heard the cliché of "crippled by the desire for perfection." These perfectionists may be unhappy with themselves, but they typically make others' lives easier by being organized. However, they can be annoying at times; annoying by being better prepared than the rest of us but still complaining.

Yet, these disorders at their worst are not easy for the individuals. They suffer personally, interpersonally, socially and professionally, in spite of trying hard to be good. They are also referred to as "neurotic" which comes from Hans Eysenck's theories of personality. He tried to explain personality types by two dimensions in the behavior including: extraversion/introversion and neuroticism. He devised scales to measure the degree of extraversion (sometimes spelled extroversion) and neuroticism and came up with different personality types based on the high or low extraversion in combination with high or low neuroticism. Neuroticism is a measure of inherent anxiety and apprehension that is reflected in one's attitude and behavior. Individuals who score high on neuroticism, understandably, are highly represented by people with anxiety disorders. High neuroticism score is correlated to or suspected to be a susceptibility factor for anxiety disorders. The personality disorders in this cluster; avoidant personality disorder, dependent personality disorder, and obsessive-compulsive personality disorder, may be

---

[4] "They may drink a cheap porridge but wash their mouths (in public) with rose water" - a Tamil proverb.

[5] The "anal" reference comes from the psychoanalytic theorists' belief that the roots of anxiety comes from the developmental stage of anal retention. They somehow equate the anxiety of a child struggling to get potty training to the anxieties or anxious behaviors of later life. There is no clear scientific basis for such thinking. But it makes a good reading. See also the chapter on psychology and psychotherapy.

associated with high score on the neuroticism scale. The common use of the word neurotic typically denotes the high neuroticism in some individual's behavior.

Avoidant Personality Disorder

There is a controversy that avoidant personality disorder is the same as, or very similar to social anxiety disorder. There is a subtle difference in the criteria, and social anxiety disorder is a very common diagnosis that you see in practice, compared to avoidant personality disorder, which you rarely see (or never, like in my case. However, it does not mean it may not exist. I could be less astute clinically to identify this or less popular to be referred a patient with this condition). Anyway, there may seem to be a significant overlap between social phobia, avoidant PD, schizoid PD, high functioning autism, and even residual schizophrenia. While schizophrenia, schizoid PD and autism lack the capacity to socialize, and may not be bothered by a lack of social life, people with social phobia and avoidant PD do desire socialization but, are struggling. In addition, the difference between social phobia or social anxiety disorder and avoidant personality disorder seems to be the associated psychopathology, such as low self-esteem, feelings of inferiority and inadequacy.

In social phobia, individuals may fear embarrassment, but in avoidant PD they tend to be too sensitive in interpersonal settings and are driven by the fear of rejection or criticism, which in turn, makes them feel inadequate, inferior and unlikable. Because of this, they avoid socialization or any interpersonal contact - especially with strangers or those whom they feel threatened by. They are shy or fearful of social situations and avoid them with a fear of disapproval or ridicule, the opposite of the histrionic PD. These individuals may not form intimate relationships, and often seek reassurance in interpersonal or work settings. They develop significant negative self-esteem, and see themselves as inadequate, inferior and unappealing. Again, the opposite of the dramatic personalities.

Dependent Personality Disorder

Individuals with dependent personality disorder (DPD) are not able to make any decision on their own and, as the name implies, are dependent on someone else to make decisions for them. If and when they need to make any decision, they feel helpless, inadequate, and seek excessive amounts of advice and reassurance. They fear being alone or to face a situation where they may be required to make a decision and avoid situations where they may be forced to make a decision. Because of their perceived need for the person they depend on, they are almost subservient to those to a point, they sacrifice all their needs and wishes to pacify the needs of the person they are dependent upon. This person may be a friend or a close family member, and people with DPD may not ever demand anything in return but for the advice and reassurance. This is because of their perceived helplessness that they cannot function without the other person. They feel uncomfortable, helpless and afraid to be alone with the dread towards having to make a decision on their own. They essentially give up their independence which brings a lot of fear and anxiety.

Obsessive Compulsive Personality Disorder

Obsessive compulsive personality disorder (OCPD) and obsessive-compulsive disorder (OCD) sound similar and may have some overlapping symptoms. But, the most important distinction is that, people with OCD are bothered by one or more specific obsession (intrusive, meaningless, disturbing, perplexing thoughts that do not have a purpose; like worrying about getting HIV from the counter-top - which is not possible). The person with OCPD may not have specific obsessions, but they would be extremely rigid and inflexible over everything in their lives, be it the process they follow to complete a project at work, budgeting money at home and following or imposing moral ethical values on themselves and their loved ones. Such an inflexibility often leads to a lack of trust of others. They are upset with others, accuse them of wrongdoing or not following the rules and alienate them. In contrast to the patients with OCD, who feel anxiety and helplessness over their undesired thoughts, people with OCPD do not feel bad about their desire or intention to be orderly. They like being organized and rigid and see others as morally weak with poor discipline.

While people with OCD may be somewhat more organized, clean and rigid than others, such a behavior defines people with OCPD. They are very preoccupied with details, rules, regulations, organization and schedule. They cannot tolerate even a little bit of give-or-take in anything they do, thus making their lives constantly unhappy and irritating. They distance others socially and interpersonally by expecting everyone to follow such a rigid lifestyle. Their rigidity with rules and regulations or processes, whether it is related to work, legal issues, personal moral or ethical values, lead them to not trust others and so, they become suspicious, monitoring, controlling or micromanaging of others. They end up trying to achieve a 100% perfectionism in everything they do, and, when they fail - which, can and does happen often, they become miserable. They often hoard things and the desire to hoard and the desire to be orderly and clean typically cause conflict. You may want a surgeon or a pilot with OCPD, or hopefully a milder form of it, but not a government regulator or a traffic police officer.

Points to consider about personality disorders
1. Personality disorder is the dysfunction of the part of the brain responsible for self-identity and interpersonal and social interaction.
2. They are as biologically based and enduring.
3. They not only cause suffering to the affected individuals, but impact others, and so society in large.
4. It is important for the bystander - the friend, family member or colleague to be aware of the personality disorder, trait or behavioral pattern.
5. There is no medication that is proven to work for any personality disorder. But comorbid conditions or symptoms can be treated with medications.
6. It is generally hard to change or modify the behavioral pattern of others and so, the idea that you can fix others is a good one for cheap novels or Bollywood movies, but not for practical reasons.
7. Similarly, it is not true that parents or upbringing makes one to develop a personality disorder. It is true that the environment - including family, street influence or the society, in general can influence our behavior and our choice of behavior but the environmental influence is very small compared to the way we are born. Such an influence is often around 10 or 20%. This is not an opinion, but based on scientific fact and genetic studies. For example, adopted children resemble the biological parents more so than adoptive parents in their behavior, attitude and temperament - even when the babies are adopted away on the day of birth. It is easy to understand if it is skin color or even intelligence, but it is difficult to understand if it is temperament or moral values and such. Imagine that the structure of the brain is genetic, and so, the scaffolding of the brain structure is biologically determined. So, for example the attitude towards religion (whether you are highly religious or not) may be biological, but what religion you choose is environmental.
8. Psychotherapy, including mentalization show some promise in educating the patients to be aware of their thought, emotion and behavior, but this area of personality disorder needs to advance a lot. It will be a very interesting and exciting area of science.

Chapter 12

Dissociative Disorders and Somatic Symptoms Disorders

The mind's modus operandi is fascinating. The complexity of the brain, and its method of operation makes the study of neuroscience, psychology and psychiatry interesting, enigmatic and alluring. The disorders described in this section are conceptually different from other disorders and so are a bit more interesting, but challenging to comprehend. These disorders involve a unique mindset which falls between full awareness and lack of insight. Patients who have these illnesses appear to understand the possibility of their symptoms not being real, but still lack control of their symptoms. It is fascinating to see patients with conversion disorder have a subtle indifference to their paralysis and it is difficult to understand how an otherwise healthy, intelligent, and logical person with hypochondriasis spend a lot of time and money on the presumed illness, with no evidence.

These illnesses are fascinating windows into the human mind, although challenging to deal with. The clinician might get frustrated with these patients, and any attempt to confront them only makes them to come back with worse symptoms. They are almost always a therapeutic challenge in the clinic. Some of these patients, like those with somatization disorder frequent primary care and may drain a lot of energy and resources. Unfortunately, the level of understanding of these illnesses is very rudimentary, and there is no clear, effective treatment.

Dissociative Disorders

Dissociation is a very interesting phenomenon. It is a temporary detachment from the reality - not a loss of reality. Dissociation occurs in a spectrum. Daydreaming or getting lost in thoughts on your drive back home are believed to be milder and benign forms of dissociation. These are considered normal, occurring on a day to day basis, without causing any problems, and may help the brain to process or consolidate information.

A more serious dissociation can occur to anyone under severe stress or trauma. In those cases, it may act as a psychological defense or coping mechanism under stress. Dissociation can occur under hypnosis or with medications like ketamine. In dissociative disorders, these occur frequently and repeatedly for no tangible purpose and can interfere with day to day functions. When the reality of the self or the world is disturbed, they are known as depersonalization/derealization Disorder. A temporary or specific loss of memory is called as dissociative Amnesia and if the amnesia includes loss of memory of the self, with an assumption of a new identity, it is known as dissociative fugue. Dissociative identity disorder or multiple personality disorder is a fragmentation of identity of the self into different streams of identity or self-consciousness.

As we all know, these illnesses are fodder for pop culture and subject for novels and movies. There is quite a bit of fascination around these diagnoses and those suffering from them, but they are not common in clinical practice, at least not the spectacular cases that make it in the news. Jason Bourne does not walk into your clinic on Monday mornings. Some even question the validity of these dissociative disorders, but this phenomenon is real but poorly understood. Dissociation occurs frequently under the influence of drugs or in association with seizures suggesting a clear biological basis. There is no proven treatment, and some of these illnesses can be chronic and disabling. Dissociative disorders occur more in women than men and are frequently associated with trauma. Etiology of these are unknown and there is no proven pharmacological treatment, although clinically, SSRIs are frequently prescribed. While some aspects of the dissociation may not be fully under control, there is a learning component to these illnesses. An individual might have a dissociation in response to stress, which offers a form of relief, reinforcing the individual to have this over and over - albeit not fully intentionally.

Depersonalization/Derealization Disorder

Depersonalization is a feeling of detachment from one's self, and derealization is a feeling of detachment from the world or the feeling that the world is unreal or dreamlike. Patients may say that their conscious self is separated from them and that they are able to watch themselves from outside. They do not lose insight, and their reality testing is intact (unlike the experience of psychosis). The patients may describe this as an out of body experience or dreaming when awake. These episodes may last for minutes, hours, or even days. They can be transient when caused by seizures, drugs or migraine, anesthesia, falling asleep, hypoxia (near death experience or part of high-altitude sickness), and can be precipitated by stress or trauma. Antidepressants such as SSRIs may help this to an extent, but current evidence is not convincing.

Dissociative Amnesia

Dissociative amnesia is an inability to recall a personal experience when there is no physiological explanation. It can be a localized memory loss about a one-time incident, a series of events (e.g. a specific trauma), systematized around a particular subject, or global - forgetting everything including personal identity. The classic amnesia seen in movies like the Bourne Identity, are about the individual forgetting everything about his or her past including their identities and personal life, is an example of generalized amnesia.

Amnesia results when an individual goes through extremely stressful event, loaded with internal conflict, like fighting an inner desire/impulse (sexual or violent), that may lead to guilt or shame. These patients are typically seen in the acute setting like emergency rooms immediately after the onset of amnesia, occurring right after the stress or trauma. They may be associated with somatoform, conversion reaction and other dissociation symptoms. Organic causes such as delirium, drug use, seizures, migraines, medications, and closed head injuries should be ruled out.

No treatment is proven to work for this. Sometimes, a lengthy interview with a goal of making the patient relax and talk freely might help them "recover" the memory. Similarly, interview under the influence of medications like sodium pentothal (Pentothal interview) or lorazepam, may bring back the memories. The idea is that these drugs make the patients reach a level of semi consciousness that relaxes and disinhibits them to a point that they open up and come out of the state of amnesia. Nonetheless, validity of the recovery and recovered memories cannot be proven. Some patients do seem to get relief, but many come back with recurring symptoms.

Dissociative Fugue

This is not included as a separate diagnosis in DSM-5 as it seems to appear almost always along with other dissociative disorders. Dissociative fugue is a global amnesia about self and the past. The individual forgets all about themselves and their past, and they may travel out of their ordinary place of living and start living somewhere else, sometime assuming a new identity.

Dissociative Identity Disorder

Previously called as multiple personality disorder, it is characterized by the presence of two or more identities or "personality states." These are typically identified as incidents of other-worldly possession across cultures. Sometimes, these can happen as isolated incidents under stress or conflict but can become chronic. The affected individual may go back and forth between the identities. The patients are not psychotic and lack conviction, but they believe and act as if he or she are different people at different times. They may refer to themselves in third-person singular or first-person plural to denote the other personality.

Considering the association with trauma and conflict, psychotherapy may help to uncover the conflict. Hypnosis might help but the practice is not scientifically validated, and the benefits are debatable. Some believe that hypnosis can cause or worsen MPD because these patients are very suggestible and may act out the other personality in the trans state. Antidepressants and anxiolytics may be helpful when there is associated depression or anxiety. PTSD symptoms, when present, may be treated with antidepressants, and alpha1 adrenergic antagonist prazosin for nightmares. Antipsychotics and antiepileptics are also used with variable success.

Somatic Symptom and Related Disorders

This is a new category in DSM-5 which includes diseases that come under psychosomatic medicine. These include somatic symptom disorder and illness anxiety disorder, previously known somatization disorder and hypochondriasis. Multiple physical complaints (usually nonspecific or vague), without a known physical abnormality, is somatic symptom disorder, and a belief or worry about having a certain specific diagnosis (like AIDS or cancer) without any evidence or symptoms is illness anxiety disorder.

This section also includes functional neurological symptom disorder, previously known as conversion disorder or hysteria and factitious disorder (Munchausen Syndrome). The interplay of psychiatry and medical illness are discussed under psychological factors affecting medical illnesses is also included here. Malingering, which is a willful act of faking an illness for a purpose is also included here.

Using the term "psychosomatic illnesses" unfortunately implies that these disorders are psychological in origin but physical in presentation, thus implying "made up" or "all in the head" of the individual. It may not be clear where the problem lies, but some of these disorders can bring forth significant distress to the individual. As mentioned in the beginning, these disorders may be frustrating to deal with. Confronting the patient, even if it in the form of reassurance, does not help and these patients move from one therapist to another when they feel challenged. It is not fair to blame the patient just because we do not understand the neuropsychological underpinnings of hypochondriasis or paralysis of the conversion disorder. There is so much unknown about how the brain works.

Somatic Symptom Disorder and Illness Anxiety Disorder

What was previously known as hypochondriasis or somatization disorder is now divided into two diseases: somatic symptom disorder (SSD) and illness anxiety disorder (IAD). Patients with SSD have multiple somatic complaints with no evidence of a physical illness and patients with IAD are preoccupied about having a specific illness with no evidence. Clinically, patients SSD present with an exaggerated complaint of physical symptoms, wanting explanation and relief. Patients with IAD seem to be more worried about having a specific illness, and complain that doctors are missing it.

Patients with SSD present with one or more physical symptoms. Some of them may be mild, and vague. They exaggerate minor discomforts and come up with variety of symptoms that do not follow any pattern. They excessively worry about some related illness, become very anxious, and spend a lot of time about the imagined illness seeking treatment. They move from one doctor to other and try any form of treatment, even when they are told there is no evidence for an illness. They remain anxious even after negative results and reassurance. This must be present for more than 6 months for a diagnosis.

Patients with IAD have a predominant preoccupation or worry about having or acquiring a major illness, often a specific illness that may not have a tangible evidence, like a hidden cancer or AIDS with a negative blood test. They may or may not present or focus on any physical symptom. They spend a lot of time getting tested or getting evaluated but would not be convinced if the test is negative. They worry about the chance of false negative and test again. They do not have thought disorder and are not illogical in other aspects of their lives. Even in the case of the argument of having the illness, they try hard to argue logically with rare examples of the diagnosis being missed or them being this one in a million rare case. They do not appear or meet the criteria for OCD or delusion or psychosis. Should last for at least 6 months for a diagnosis.

Both these disorders can be episodic or chronic. The treatment includes psychotherapy, group therapy and medications focused on associated symptoms like depression and anxiety. The severity of this illness varies from a mild occurrence following stressful life event or chronic to a point, some patients spend their entire life savings on testing, retesting and going to different doctors and specialists. Approaching these patients is tricky. If you confront or bluntly report that they are OK and it is all in the head, they would become defensive, present with more symptoms, or go to a different doctor. But it is also not a good idea to play along and behave like they have a serious illness. A patient, simple, nonjudgmental discussion about the various possibilities and suggestion of the likelihood of a psychosomatic illness may help the patient consider the diagnosis. They are more accepting when it comes from another patient with same condition. Hence, group therapy with people with similar diagnoses help.

Functional Neurological Symptom Disorder

The subject was 13 or 14 in high school. He was placed in a dilemma to choose between a boot camp or a family vacation. Choosing the vacation over the boot camp is a loss of face, because he needed to assert himself by enduring the tough camp. He signed up for the camp, but as the departure date came, he fell ill. He initially thought he was having a fever then sincerely believed that he had the flu as he started experiencing the symptoms of flu, but he had doubts. He was advised not to go to the camp with the fever, and so he "reluctantly" went with his family on vacation. After a day in bed, while on vacation, the flu magically disappeared. He was confused; he "knew" he was not faking the flu, but he was not sure. He wondered whether he made his body get the flu, the real one. He was also wondering whether he really got the flu as a coincidence or whether he brought forth or caused it willfully.

In this example, the patient suspected that the symptoms may not be real but started believing it at some point. He was worried about the shame of chickening out from the boot camp, causing an internal conflict. But when he started believing his illness, his anxiety or shame disappeared, and the internal conflict resolved. This is called as the "primary gain." The attention and sympathy he got from the teachers and family is the "secondary gain." La belle indifference is the lack of concern of the patient. Patients with "paralysis" and "blindness" may not appear to be adequately or appropriately concerned. Identification is another attribute of such conversions where patients emulate the condition of someone they know or someone important (a celebrity) who is getting a lot of attention from a certain illness.

Conversion symptoms are almost always preceded by a personal psychological conflict. A range of neurological symptoms can occur including; paralysis, tremors, seizures, paresthesias, numbness, as well as blindness, deafness or falls. The patients do not have consistent neurological signs and symptoms that point to a known illness. Paralysis may not be accompanied by adequate atrophy, bed sores or heightened reflexes. Distraction may reduce the symptoms like tremor or weakness. An "unconscious" patient may actively resist opening of the eyes.

Functional Neurological Symptom Disorder is very common and is reported to constitute 5-15% of psychiatric consultations in a general hospital (25-30 % in Veterans Administration hospital). They are more common in women. Depression and anxiety may be associated. Once again, confrontation of these patients might make them worse and they may come up with more symptoms, so is ignoring them. Long term psychotherapy and treatment of associated depression and anxiety or other symptoms are warranted. Identification of the conflict and resolution would be a key issue in psychotherapy.

Factitious Disorder

Also known as Munchausen's syndrome, is an unusual illness in which individuals frequently risk their lives to become patients. They feign, exaggerate and often induce, an illness to gain admission to a hospital. At times, they may inflict painful, deforming and life-threatening conditions. These patients often have a background in healthcare (nurses, physicians) or are closely related or associated with health care professionals. With some basic knowledge of medicine, and pathology, they may ingest drugs or chemicals to induce sickness, or inject contaminated material into their veins to produce septicemia. When they do this to someone else, typically someone dependent on them like a child, it is called Munchausen syndrome by proxy.

The cause of factitious disorder is unknown. No biological basis or genetic pattern has been established. Patients may have stress, conflict, and poor self-image issues. They may learn, or get the idea, when one of their relatives gets sick or as healthcare workers, they may come across some dramatic patients or illnesses that gained a lot of attention and slowly develop the habit of afflicting similar illness to get to the hospital and gain attention. There is no proven treatment and the issue of the safety of the patient, as well as the affected in case of factitious disorder by proxy, is the main concern along with medico-legal issues and child protection.

Pseudocyesis

Pseudocyesis or phantom pregnancy is a strange condition where the patients develop all signs and symptoms of pregnancy without being pregnant. Women sometimes develop this under internal or external pressure to become pregnant. They would have all the symptoms of pregnancy including amenorrhea, breast tenderness, morning sickness and a distention of the abdomen, which is actually filled with gas (the distention disappears under general anesthesia). Pseudo pregnancy has been reported in husbands or partners known as Couvade syndrome or sympathetic pregnancy. It is also found in other mammals.

Psychological Factors Affecting Medical Illnesses

A number of medical illnesses are affected by psychiatric comorbidity and are influenced by psychological factors. An increased anxiety before surgery is known to make the surgery and the postoperative recovery more complicated and protracted. Mortality from coronary artery disease doubles in the presence of depression. Psychiatric illnesses and stress influence the outcome of cancer, infection, surgery and complicate neurodegenerative disorders such as Parkinson's disease and dementia. As the understanding of the interplay of the body and mind improves, it has become clear that psychological factors can lead to somatic symptoms, and psychiatric comorbidity frequently causes, or worsens physical illnesses. It is prudent for all physicians to be aware of the psychological mechanisms and psychiatric illnesses influencing the physical illnesses.

The idea that stress causing, contributing or worsening a physical illness is not new, but the extent this spans to a range of organ systems and diseases is impressive. Type A personality and its relationship to coronary artery disease is such a popular idea that heart attack following stress is a common plot twist in dramatic movies and soap operas. People also refer to a certain laxity of the colon or gastrointestinal tract under stress or fear (colloquially referred as "shitting in my pants"), often in a symbolic manner, but one can be sure that such a thing happened to us at some point.

Stress

Stress in itself is a very interesting topic. Stress is the body's response to a stressor. Stress influences body's normal physiological and psychological functioning. The bodily response to both positive and negative stress is similar. For example, marriage and childbirth are considered some of the most stressful life events, even though they are positive. Walter Cannon (1871-1945) demonstrated activation of the autonomic nervous system that prepares the body to handle stress by increasing the blood pressure, heart rate and cardiac output. He called this "fight-or-flight" response, as the animal prepares to either fight the danger or run for safety. Although we do not need to run from the lion in the modern age of cellphones, zoos, and fast foods, we still respond to stressful situations in a manner that prepares for us to fight the lion. In addition to the cardiac changes, our breathing increases oxygen intake, our attention becomes acute, vision becomes more focused, pain, hunger, and other bodily issues become less apparent and less important. Hans Selye (1907-1982) studied stress response extensively and proposed a theory called "general adaptation syndrome" which included an alarm reaction, stage of resistance, and a stage of exhaustion.

Stress response is supposed to be a protective and a survival mechanism which may be less relevant in the modern society. However, exaggerated or chronic stress responses appear to cause or worsen several diseases from coronary artery disease to skin problems, in addition to be a problem in itself. The body's response includes activation of the noradrenergic system in the locus coeruleus, causing release of catecholamines in the brain. In addition, serotonin, dopamine, GABA and NMDA receptors may also be involved. Corticotropin-releasing factor (CRF) as a neurotransmitter on its own has been implicated as a mediator of stress and has been a target for experimental medications for depression. CRF, secreted in the hypothalamus is responsible for most of the stress response of hormones that has further downstream effect.

CRF activates secretion of adrenocorticotropic hormone (ACTH) in the anterior pituitary, which, in turn, floods the body with glucocorticoids (corticosteroids) from the adrenal glands. Glucocorticoids promote glucose use, and increase cardiac activity, as mentioned above. They also slow growth and suppress reproduction and immunity. Although steroids suppress immunity, stress is known to activate immunity, and many autoimmune disorders are activated or worsen under stress. It is believed that there are other molecules similar to ACTH that increase the net glucocorticoids in the body (known as secretagogues) that also may play a role in stress response.

Stress affect people differently. Some may respond with cardiac symptoms while others may respond with GI tract. Wonder why we feel like we need to go to the bathroom more often during exam days? The specific pattern of bodily response to stress may be genetic or learned from the individual's past experience. They also vary depending upon the time of one's life, a perception of inevitability and so on. For example, a common catastrophe like natural disasters are handled differently from individual setbacks. Stress or stressful life events can also make one stronger and more resilient (what doesn't kill you makes you stronger). Among the life events death of the spouse is considered as the most stressful with a score of 100 (marriage is 50, divorce is 73, being fired from job is 43 and death of a family member is rated at 63).

There is a long list of illnesses spanning across several organ systems that are affected by psychological factors and a detailed description of each disease is beyond the scope of this book. A number of gastrointestinal diseases including globus (lump in the throat), dyspepsia, constipation, diarrhea, pain (chest, abdomen and anorectal area), and irritable bowel syndrome are known to be affected by stress and they have a high incidence of comorbid anxiety and depression. Peptic ulcer is sometimes found to be associated with stress, but evidence is not convincing. Anxiety and stress influence the presentation and symptomatology in ulcerative colitis and Crohn's disease.

Type A personality (being driven, angry, impatient, task oriented, hostility and negative emotions) is associated with increased risk of Coronary Artery Disease (CAD). Presence of depression almost doubles post CAD morbidity and mortality. Stress and anxiety worsen arrhythmias and hypertension. Psychosocial intervention including psychoeducation, social support, stress management and relaxation lead to better post CAD outcome with lower BP, heart rate, and lower cholesterol. Patients who did not receive this kind of support are found to have 70% more mortality and 84% more repeat cardiac events.

Asthma mimics panic attacks, and about 30% of patients with asthma have an anxiety disorder. It is understandable that an acute attack of asthma, with a hunger for air and a fear for life, can make one learn to become anxious. Relaxation, and behavioral therapy, and treatment for anxiety can help both anxiety and asthma symptoms. Patients with hyperthyroidism frequently present with anxiety, irritability, dysphoria or euphoria, and patients with hypothyroidism can present with severe depression, memory loss, and anxiety. Cushing's syndrome can cause classic panic attacks, anxiety, and depression. Hypercortisolism can present with anxiety, depression or mania.

Psychological factors and stress can worsen the symptoms of atopic dermatitis (Eczema), psoriasis, psychogenic excoriation, pruritus ani, pruritus vulvae, hyperhidrosis and urticaria. Management of rheumatoid arthritis, systemic lupus erythematosus, fibromyalgia, low back pain, migraines and headaches should include psychosocial aspects. Identification of anxiety, depression and other comorbid conditions as well as a general education for stress management should be part of the treatment regimen in managing any chronic medical illnesses. However, this aspect of patient care is often ignored.

Chapter 13

Dementia

"My husband of 48 years is leaving me. Ever so slowly... He is sitting just next to me, but he is not there. Not anymore. He smiles at me but has no clue why. He knows nothing about what he did, what he has, or what he wants. He is losing me and losing himself and he does not know it. Unlike him, I am so aware of all this. Why can't I get the dementia?"

Dementia is a major public health challenge of the 21st century. About one in 4 individuals above the age of 85 have dementia, and one in three elderly eventually die from it. Incidence of dementia increases as we get older, from 5% among 71-79-year-old to 37.4% among 90 or older. It is estimated that there are 46.8 million people with dementia in the world. The societal cost of dementia in the USA is believed to be $159 to $215 billion with each patient costing between $41,000 to $56,000. Dementia causes a significant burden to the caregiver, in terms of time, emotion and money.

Dementia is not a single disease. It is a syndrome characterized by a decline in cognitive functioning caused by various conditions including Alzheimer's disease (about 60 to 80% of all cases), vascular dementia (10%), other types including Lewy body dementia, and frontotemporal dementia. Dementia can also result from chronic traumatic brain injury, substance use, alcohol use, medication use, HIV, Prion disease, Huntington's Chorea, Parkinson's disease, and other medical problems.

The DSM 5 does not use the word "dementia." Instead, it is referred as neurocognitive disorders (NCD), (major NCD for dementia and amnesic disorder and mild NCD for mild cognitive disorders). It also moved the emphasis from impairment in memory and expanded the cognitive domains to learning and memory, complex attention, executive function, language, perceptual motor function, and social cognition. There is a requirement of interference with daily activities, and exclusion of delirium and other medical conditions for a diagnosis.

Clinical Features

Cognitive deficits start slow and decline over time. The diagnosis becomes obvious when the condition is advanced, but it may be difficult to identify in the early stages. For example, a subtle cognitive decline in a high functioning individual can go unnoticed for some time, and individuals who are in demanding jobs may show a decline in performance before cognitive deficits become obvious. Some retirees with minimal demands in day to day life may manage with significant cognitive deficits and may go unnoticed and undiagnosed until late.

Significant forgetfulness is the telltale sign of early dementia, but patients may present with decline in other areas of cognition. It is not uncommon for a patient to exhibit socially inappropriate behavior as an early symptom. Occasional troubles in memory or a mild decline in cognition may not be a problem but the key here is decline and the degree of decline. A steady decline from previous level of functioning should alert patients and caregivers to the possibility of dementia.

In early stages, patients may recognize their cognitive decline but, often, they are not fully aware of it as the insight gets compromised. While they still have some awareness of the deficits, they try to conceal them by rationalizing or covering with anger, jokes or sarcasm and complain of being mentally tired or disinterested. They try to compensate by working harder, being more detail oriented, and organized.

Initially, cognitively demanding tasks like keeping track of finances or learning something new may be difficult but, as the deficit progresses even remembering basic things like daily chores become difficult. As the mental process becomes more and more affected, their speech and ability to express themselves are impaired and their conversation becomes less and less informative. They try hard not to make mistakes by not committing to something or by avoiding details. For example, if you ask, "What type of work am I doing here?" they would say "You are here taking care of things," answering in a general manner. They get frustrated with the lack of knowledge and try to fill in things that they think are missing (confabulation) or stick to what they know. They attempt to compensate by changing the subject, divert with a joke, or hide behind anger and agitation. They have problems learning or understanding new concepts, and impairment in logical thinking, reasoning, problem solving and judgment. Their speech becomes vague, lacking details, monotonous, repetitive (perseveration), imprecise or circumstantial. Orientation to person, time and place will be affected as the disease progresses. Their personalities change. They may become disinhibited and behave inappropriately or become withdrawn or anxious. A number of psychiatric problems including psychosis, depression, and anxiety disorders can occur. They can develop neurological complications including apraxia, aphasia, agnosia and seizures.

Types of Dementia

Dementia of the Alzheimer's type (AD), is the most common type of dementia. AD is a neurodegenerative disease, and a brain with Alzheimer's disease appears shrunken. However, a shrunken brain is not diagnostic or specific to AD, meaning even normal people can have a shrunken brain. The brain does shrink with old age, although not as much as in AD. In AD, there is tissue damage, neuronal cell death and loss of neuronal connections leading to the loss of mass. The degree of degeneration is related to accumulation of plaques and tangles.

Plaques are clumps of a protein called beta-amyloid and are found between the cells. The plaques or beta-amyloid clumps interfere with neuronal communication and may be toxic to the cells causing inflammation and destruction. The neurofibrillary tangles are formed by the breakdown of a protein called tau protein. Tau helps keep the intracellular transportation system intact. With its breakdown, and formation of the tangles, the cells become incapable of feeding or operating themselves, resulting in neuronal death. The amyloid hypothesis or accumulation of amyloid is believed to be the cause of AD, but this is sometimes disputed. AD runs in families and several genes including APOE4 (apolipoprotein) and a few others have been implicated in its pathology. APOE4 seems to interfere with the clearance of beta amyloid. There are new treatments using monoclonal antibodies of the amyloid in the testing phase.

Vascular Dementia

This is the second most common cause of dementia or NCD, and at times referred to as multi infarct dementia. As its name implies, this dementia is caused by a sequence of small strokes or infarcts in the brain. The risk factors for cerebrovascular disease include hypertension, diabetes, smoking, high cholesterol, cardiovascular disease and old age. Sometimes, the amyloid plaques from AD can damage blood vessels and cause a stroke that worsens the dementia. The symptoms and signs vary depending upon the area of the brain involved. A typical feature of vascular dementia is a stepwise pattern in the cognitive decline and a sudden loss of cognitive function is noted immediately after each stroke. A popular scale known as Hachinski Ischemic scale is used to list the risk factors for vascular dementia. A score of 7 or above is indicative of vascular dementia. Binswanger's disease is a form of multi-infarct dementia, which is also referred as subcortical arteriosclerotic encephalopathy. It results from multiple small infarcts caused by atherosclerosis of small arteries feeding the white matter. A classic sign of this illness is psychomotor slowing. The patient may take an inordinate amount of time to complete a task like buttoning the shirt or writing his or her name.

Hachinski Ischemic Scale	
Feature	Score
Abrupt onset	2
Stepwise deterioration	1
Fluctuating course	2
Nocturnal confusion	1
Relative preservation of personality	1
Depression	1
Somatic complaints	1
Emotional incontinence	1
History of strokes	2
Evidence of atherosclerosis	1
Focal neurological symptoms	2
Focal neurological signs	2
History or presence of hypertension	1

Lewy Body Dementia

Lewy body dementia (Dementia with Lewy Bodies - DLB) is the third most common type of dementia. It is named after Frederic H. Lewy who discovered the dementia while working with Alzheimer. The Lewy bodies consist of alpha synuclein protein. Patients with Lewy body dementia may be differentiated from Alzheimer's dementia by the presence of visual hallucinations, Parkinsonian symptoms including rigidity, tremors or bradykinesia (difficulty initiating movements), REM sleep related problems and mood problems such as depression. DLB acts like Parkinson's disease because the dopaminergic neurons are involved. It also affects cholinergic neurons, similar to AD.

Frontotemporal Lobar Degeneration

Frontotemporal lobar degeneration is a rare degenerative disease, affecting the frontal and temporal lobes where accumulation of tau particles and another protein called TDP-43 results in shrinkage of these lobes. Considering the variability of the involvement and the location of the damage, a variety of symptoms including personality change, behavioral problems, speech and language problems, and movement disorders occur. It used to be called Pick's disease and the clumps of tau particles used to be called as Pick's bodies.

Prion Disease

Prion is a transmissible protein that has no DNA or RNA but behaves like a virus, spreading in the brain tissue. Jacob-Creutzfeldt disease is the most famous example. The prion spreads from infected cows (Mad Cow disease). Other examples of prion related diseases are scrapie, a disease of the sheep, kuru, a brain degenerative disorder and Gerstmann-Straussler syndrome, a familial progressive dementia. The prion disease cause spongiform degeneration of the brain, and they frequently have ataxia and myoclonus along with dementia.

Other causes for dementia include normal pressure hydrocephalus, Parkinson's disease, Huntington's disease, HIV infection, substance use, alcohol use, traumatic brain injury, and other medical conditions. Some of these causes including hypothyroidism, vitamin B12 deficiency, neurosyphilis, and Lyme disease are treatable and so the dementia can be reversed, or stopped in its progress. A thorough evaluation to rule out the reversible causes should be part of the treatment.

The diagnosis of dementia is essentially clinical, and it can only be confirmed by pathological examination of the brain tissue. Neuroimaging such as CT scan and MRI are not diagnostic for AD, but are helpful to rule out other causes (infarcts, tumors, prion diseases). CT and MRI would show the "shrinkage" and may be useful in assessing the progress of the disease. PET (Positron Emission Tomography) imaging can detect and measure beta amyloid and tau particles. They are also not necessarily diagnostic, but progression or recovery can be measured. CSF measure of these proteins is also used occasionally. At this point, investigations are underway to identify an easily detectable biomarkers to diagnose cognitive deficits early.

Treatment

There is no cure or treatment to reverse or stop the progression of the neurodegenerative process. The available treatments help improve cognition or just mask the cognitive deficits of dementia. Cholinesterase inhibitors increase the level of acetylcholine by inhibiting the enzyme acetylcholinesterase. Acetylcholine is a key neurotransmitter for cognitive functions including memory. The degenerative process in dementia destroys the neurons and neuronal connections interfering with acetylcholine metabolism. These medications temporarily increase the level of acetylcholine and improve cognition for a short time. They have annoying side effects, including nausea, vomiting, diarrhea, muscle cramps, cardiac side effects, headache and insomnia. These drugs do not slow the progression of the dementia and their utility in mild cognitive deficit is debatable, considering the side effects. However, they are used widely and frequently. The acetylcholinesterase inhibitors include tetrahydroaminoacridine (Tacrine), donepezil, rivastigmine, metrifonate and galantamine.

Memantine is an NMDA receptor antagonist. It is believed to reduce the excitotoxic effects of glutamate. Again, memantine improves cognition but does not slow or stop the progress of neurodegeneration. These drugs help gain "a few months" in the progressive decline of cognitive function. Newer treatments include monoclonal antibodies for beta amyloid. The idea is to get rid of the amyloid that accumulates in the brain. Some early results of this approach are disappointing, but it is believed that they would be helpful in mild to moderate cases. Clinical trials are underway. But, there are doubts that amyloid itself may not be the reason for dementia.

Patients with dementia, or any degenerative disease can develop various psychiatric symptoms and syndromes including depression, anxiety or psychosis, and should be treated appropriately. Patients with agitation or confusion are frequently treated with antipsychotics, or benzodiazepines. Behavioral problems including agitation, verbal or physical aggression, wandering, intrusiveness, uncooperativeness, disinhibition and sexually inappropriate behavior etc., are major issues in managing these patients. Reassurance, redirection, with structured and routine activities help. Safety is the predominant issue and patients may need to be protected from falls and injuries. An evaluation for worsening behavior should include, an assessment of comorbid conditions, medications, psychiatric issues and other medical issues. Agitation is typically treated by small dose of benzodiazepines and/or antipsychotics. It is important to keep in mind that sedative drugs increase chance of fall and fractures. It is important to rule out delirium (see below) which worsens agitation. Caregiver burnout because of these behavioral problems is also common.

Delirium

Delirium is a common disorder and a frequent reason for psychiatric consultation in general hospitals, where 14% to 24% of patients are estimated to experience delirium. 6% to 56% of postoperative patients and a staggering 87% of the ICU patients develop delirium. Delirium occurs in 60% of individuals in nursing homes and 83% of end of life patients.

Delirium is not a disease. It is a syndrome resulting from a compromise in the homeostasis of the brain, usually from multiple physiological abnormalities. It can be caused by a single problem such as epilepsy or alcohol withdrawal, or a combination of risk factors. The chance of delirium increases as the risk factors increase. For example, the chance of postoperative delirium increases depending upon the stress or complexity of the surgery, tissue damage, blood loss, electrolyte imbalance, infection, pain, insomnia, narcotics and other medications besides the age of the patient. The elderly are more susceptible for delirium, especially if they have additional risk factors like dementia or stroke. Old age, preexisting brain damage such as dementia, nutritional deficiency, malignancies, cerebrovascular disease, infection, alcohol or drug use, and sensory deprivation, increase the odds of developing delirium.

The hallmark of delirium is impaired attention. The patients have difficulty in directing, sustaining or shifting attention to any task. They have difficulty answering questions or engaging in a conversation. They may seem listless, confused with a wandering and fleeting attention towards seemingly irrelevant things. As a result, they may not be able to process where they are, what they are doing or even who they are, leading to confusion and disorientation. In addition, they may also have cognitive deficits, memory impairment, language problems, visuospatial difficulties, and hallucinations. The confusion, disorientation and lack of attention leads to significant behavioral problems. Patients in the ICU may try to pull the IV, catheters or endotracheal intubation, often leading to complications.

Delirium has a waxing and waning presentation, with confusion and agitation varying by the hour, and getting worse in the evening (sundowning), with lucid intervals in between. Quite often, even when the patient seems clear, they may be disoriented or have difficulties with attention. Simple questions on orientation, short term memory or simple bedside tests for attention (asking them to spell the word "world" (or any word) backwards or asking them to subtract 7s from 100), would reveal the impairment in attention and are useful in the diagnosis.

Delirium usually lasts for a few days, rarely more than a week, and gets better as the underlying condition improves. Occasional patients may have chronic delirium, but prolonged delirium is an indication of an unresolved underlying cause and may lead to seizures, coma or death. Patients in delirium frequently have visual hallucinations, exhibit perseveration (answering the previous question or lingering on the topic of the first question) along with agitation and anxiety.

Although the delirium develops suddenly, patients may exhibit some subtle symptoms and signs a day or two before the onset of delirium including: preoccupation, apprehension, anxiety, restlessness, sleep disturbances, nightmares and brief hallucinations. Along with these symptoms, level of consciousness, arousal and sleep are usually impaired. They may be hyperactive with heightened arousal, or hypoactive and drowsy. They do not sleep well and may wander at night, confused. Besides being a sign of delirium, poor sleep can precipitate or exaggerate delirium.

Management of patients with delirium includes, safety and the treatment of the underlying cause. They benefit from a small dose of antipsychotics such as haloperidol 2 to 5 mg, especially when they are hallucinating. Benzodiazepines (lorazepam 1mg) are very useful in agitation and insomnia. However, it is important to keep in mind that some medications are major contributors to delirium, especially among patients in the ICU or postoperative wards. Narcotic painkillers and drugs with anticholinergic effect contribute to the delirium and it is not uncommon to see patients improve within a day when the narcotics are stopped.

Chapter 14

Child Psychiatry

Symptoms of mental illnesses such as psychosis or depression are conceptually adult in nature as they may need a fully formed psyche. Small children may not be able to express their nihilism in an eloquent manner and may not have developed the logical reasoning, which is affected in schizophrenia. When children are sad or anxious, they may respond with fear, anger or behavioral problems. These adult illnesses are rare in children below 10 but as they grow, they begin to exhibit adult symptoms and by the teenage years, almost all mental disorders become diagnosable. In addition to the "adult illnesses" showing up early in children, a lot of children who would eventually develop mental illnesses as adults, exhibit premorbid symptoms and signs. For example, personality disorders are diagnosed at the age of 18, but teens show signs long before their 18th birthday. In this section, disorders exclusive in children are discussed.

These include neurodevelopmental disorders, resulting from an impaired development of the brain. Many of these disorders are more common among children born prematurely or with low birth weight. Complications during pregnancy or delivery, or any interference, insult or injury to the normal prenatal development of the brain increase the probability of these disorders. The neurodevelopmental disorders of childhood include: Autism Spectrum Disorders, Attention Deficit/Hyperactivity Disorder, Intellectual Disabilities, Motor Disorders, Specific Learning Disorders and Communication Disorders.

Autism Spectrum Disorders (ASD)

Interestingly, Eugen Bleuler who coined the word schizophrenia was also behind the use of the word autism (in German, Autismus). Initially, he meant autism was one of the four core symptoms of schizophrenia along with associational disturbances, affective flattening, and ambivalence (so called Bleuler's 4 As). He meant autism in this context as living with oneself or intensely self-absorbed (Auto = self). Later this word was used exclusively for the childhood disorder autism in which the individual has significant deficits in social communication and social interaction; thus, just living with oneself.

Autism is a fairly common disorder affecting 1 in 68 children (4 times more common in boys than girls) and is being diagnosed more often these days, possibly because of an increase in awareness, and a broader diagnostic category. Understandably, autism is devastating for the young parents, and evokes very strong emotional response that may be behind the unsubstantiated rumors connecting autism to vaccination[1].

Autism was not well recognized until mid-part of 20th century. Henry Maudsley in 1897 recognized the developmental delays in children but those days individuals with symptoms of autism were identified as having psychosis. In 1943 Leo Kanner published a seminal paper titled "Autistic Disturbances of Affective Contact" that defined the current diagnosis and the concept of autism. Kanner, an Austrian physician, a cardiologist by training, emigrated to USA after World War I, happened to get a job in a state hospital in South Dakota. With no training in psychiatry or pediatrics, and just by sheer interest, he became the first "child psychiatrist" in the USA. He also published the first child psychiatry textbook in English in 1935. He is considered as the father of American child psychiatry. He described the symptoms of autism in a clear, complete and comprehensive manner, and called it "infantile autism." His characterization of autism includes: disturbances in social behavior (desired aloneness), impairment in language and communication, anxious and obsessive desire for sameness, and starting very early (infants not leaning forward when picked up). He differentiated this condition from schizophrenia by how autistic children fail to establish an ability to form a social relationship, as opposed to patients with schizophrenia who seem to lose the capacity they had earlier.

Diagnosis and Clinical Features

The DSM-5 simplified the criteria for autism from DSM IV, which used "pervasive developmental disorder" as a diagnosis moving more or less toward Kanner's original description. The simplification of DSM-5 includes everything from infantile autism, childhood autism, Kanner's autism, high-functioning autism, PDD not otherwise speci-

---

1 Lancet published a paper in 1998 and later retracted it in 2010, that claimed that MMR vaccines may cause autism. There is no proof of connection between vaccination and autism.

fied, childhood disintegrative disorder, and Asperger's disorder. Such a simplification emphasizes the lack of knowledge of the pathophysiology of ASD to differentiate between them.

The DSM criteria includes deficits in social interaction and social communication (criterion A), and restricted, repetitive patterns of behavior, interests or activities (criterion B). These symptoms must be present from birth (criterion C) and the criterion D requires the necessary impairment for a disorder. DSM-5 also differentiates this condition into mild, moderate and severe based on how much support the patient needs. The symptoms vary in severity depending upon age, training, intellectual and language impairment.

The classic manifestation of autism is an impairment in social/emotional reciprocity; the "give and take," or the ability to go back and forth, in a social interaction. They do not understand others' emotions adequately or appropriately and lack the skills to react with appropriate emotional or behavioral responses. They may not initiate a social interaction or fail to respond properly when initiated by others. They lack the ability to emotionally join others by sharing the interest, enthusiasm or affect, required to enjoy the company of others. They lack nonverbal communication skills such as body language, eye contact, gestures, and the capacity to integrate verbal and nonverbal communication. They have deficits in understanding, developing or maintaining social relationships, and they do not comprehend the contextual differences in relationships. Such a deficit in social interaction may range from a simple social awkwardness or inappropriateness, to a complete lack of social behavior. The severity of the deficit is exacerbated when they also have language and intellectual disability.

Criterion B requires two of the four items in the restricted and repetitive pattern of behavior: repetitive body movements, insistence of the sameness, fixation on something unusual, and abnormally high or low reaction to sensory input. The repetitive motor movements can be tic like purposeless movements (eye blinking), or speech - utterance of the same word over and over, and purposeless and repetitive use of objects such as flipping the pen cap or twirling buttons on the shirt. The insistence on sameness is reflected in their difficulty to adopt to changes in their surroundings or routine. They may not be doing every single thing in a particular, repetitive manner but they are inflexible about certain specific things in their lives. This could be eating on the same plate, or the food being arranged in a certain way (with no obvious or understandable rule), same bed sheet no matter where they go, same seat in the bus etc. Any change in the routine would result in protest that can sometimes turn into a major behavioral problem. They show highly fixated and restricted interest; for no particular reason, they may collect a toy of a certain kind, or even objects that are apparently meaningless to others. They may show hyper or hypo sensitivity to sensory stimuli. They may react in extreme manner to some sensory stimuli (like wanting to hear train sirens repeatedly or being intolerant to the sprinkler sound) or preoccupied with some lights, texture or other sensory stimuli.

Causes

Autism may be caused by various etiologies leading to a single pathology, or it may have several different etiopathological pathways resulting in similar symptoms (say, like seizures). There is evidence that the brain is affected very early, around the time of conception, or during the early months of pregnancy. For example, exposure to a number of teratogens (agents that affect the development of the fetus) in the early months of pregnancy, including heavy metals, solvents, diesel fumes, pesticides, alcohol, smoking, illicit drugs and even stress is associated with ASD. Congenital rubella, phenylketonuria or complications during labor are associated with autism. However, there is no evidence that vaccination results in autism or ASD and the brain abnormalities associated with autism start long before the vaccination is given.

Autism runs in families and so has a strong genetic basis, with the heritability estimated at up to 0.9 (meaning 90% of the susceptibility is inherited[2]). Like many mental illnesses, it is probably polygenetic, meaning multiple genes are likely to be involved in the pathophysiology of the syndrome. The brain abnormalities in ASD are not well understood. A number of brain abnormalities including larger brain size, increased number of neurons or neuronal connections or erroneous connections, have been proposed, but no clear abnormality has been identified. ASD is extremely variable in presentation in terms of the range and severity of the symptoms, suggesting the possibility that there may not be a single cause or a single detectable brain abnormality.

Treatment

There is no proven biological therapy or medication for ASD. Any associated problems such as seizures, depression or psychosis need to be treated appropriately. Behavioral problems associated with ASD are sometimes managed by antidepressants such as SSRIs or antipsychotics such as haloperidol, risperidone or aripiprazole. Considering the ex-

---

2 Say, for example if one is measuring a certain trait (personality or eye color) and its variation among individuals, these statistical measures determine how much of any variation in that trait is heritable vs environmentally decided. 0 would be purely environmental and 1 would be entirely determined by the genes. Something like skin color can be assumed to be mostly heritable. Autism seems to be highly heritable.

treme variability in the presentation and associated disability (intellectual and language), it is difficult to study any treatment method, especially the psychosocial intervention. However, it seems that the training, education and behavioral intervention helps these children, especially when started early. Their ability to learn and improve also depends on the level of underlying disability. But it is important to know that almost all children with ASD can learn, train and improve to an extent.

Attention Deficit/Hyperactivity Disorder (ADD and ADHD)

ADHD is one of the most controversial and contentious diagnoses in psychiatry. The opinions can be extreme between the believers and non-believers, at times taking a religious fervor. There are several possible reasons for this: The distinction between normal and abnormal is somewhat vague, which is true in many psychiatric diagnoses but almost anyone who reads this can identify with several symptoms of ADHD, the criteria are subjective, and appear a bit flexible. Non-believers question the validity of the diagnosis and believers see ADHD in everyone. Some consider the treatment with stimulants as drug abuse, and an unfair performance enhancing technique, but others see that the idea of performance enhancement itself is a good thing, and feel that such an opportunity should be given to everyone by making stimulants available without a prescription.

The stimulants are addictive and unsafe, which evokes strong emotions. A lot of people knowingly abuse the stimulants and use the diagnosis to rationalize and justify, but, some patients who might actually benefit from stimulants refuse to take them because of the addiction potential. The distinction between treating a disease and enhancing the performance in otherwise normal people is somewhat nebulous in ADHD. General public, experts, celebrities and media have strong opinions about ADHD and its treatment, making it a cultural phenomenon.

There is even controversy or discrepancy in the prevalence of ADHD, which is estimated to be around 5% using DSM criteria, but only 1% using ICD 10 criteria! There is an undeniable bias from patients, parents and clinicians on both sides. However, it is clear that the diagnosis is overused and "treatment" or use of stimulants is excessive; about 20% of young adults in some parts of United States use prescription stimulants.

Attention is a brain function influenced by a range of factors. More or less like pain, attention or attentional impairment can be caused by a number of day-to-day events. Sleep is a major factor; poor sleep impairs attention, concentration and focus, and a better night's sleep helps us stay focused in the next day. Sedating medications such as diphenhydramine (Benadryl), alcohol, lack of exercise, and nutrition can all influence the level of attention. Caffeine, a stimulant that improves attention, is the most commonly used drug in the world. Americans consume about 400 million cups of coffee every day. Worldwide, 8.5 million metric tons of coffee and 4.7 million metric tons of tea, enough for about a trillion cups of coffee and 2.5 trillion cups of tea is produced annually, inundating the humankind with stimulants[3]. Consumption of so much stimulants clearly indicates our desire or need for a boost in our focus. But for the addiction potential, and the harms of smoking, nicotine would also join tea and coffee in popularity. So, stimulant market is huge. If only the ADHD definition is stretched a bit and if the stimulants are safer than what they are, this would be a great business opportunity.

A combination or parental pressure, clinician bias, patients' willingness to identify a "disorder" for their attentional shortcomings, has influenced the popularity of this diagnosis. The patient is happy to receive a performance enhancing controlled substance, legally, without guilt, and the doctor is happy to see a satisfied patient, resulting in a perfect storm. It is estimated that 20% of young adults in America take prescription stimulants, and they are popular "street drugs" during exams. Even if the prevalence is 5%, a 20% consumption means three out of four who take stimulants do not have the disease and if the prevalence is 1%, 19 out of 20 or 95% of those who take stimulants do not have the disease. Interestingly, some of the individuals who actually have ADHD do not want to take stimulants because of the addiction potential.

On the other hand, relatively poor attention or some distractibility may not always be a bad thing. Creativity is associated with some distractibility and some neuroscientists think that distractibility is normal, and our brains are built for being distracted, so that we can be attentive of the lurking dangers. There is an evolutionary basis for the benefit of short attention span. Long textbooks and tasks requiring intense attention (like day long schools and classes) are modern inventions that the ancient brain is trying hard to accommodate (thus, so much coffee!). Yet, ADHD and ADD are real and the sufferer struggles with the demands of school and day to day life.

Clinical features and diagnosis

Despite the controversy, ADHD is a real disease and it is unmistakable in severely affected children. Boys are affected more often than

---

[3] (Spoiler alert!) Those of you who are fans of the famous comic series Asterix and Obelix may remember that the druid brews a magic potion that gives Asterix invincibility (Obelix fell in the cauldron as a baby and so he does not need it). In Asterix in Britain, the druid runs out of his magic ingredients for the potion and so he improvises with some local ingredient - tea.

girls. The DSM requires a persistent pattern of inattention and hyperactivity that starts early (DSM requires age 12), but the symptoms are generally apparent by age 4, present in two or more settings (home, classroom, clinic), and should clearly be interfering normal functioning. For inattention, the diagnosis requires the presence of at least 6 out of the 9 symptoms: 1) failing to pay attention to details or making careless mistakes, 2) difficulty sustaining attention, 3) mind wandering or inability to pay attention while talking, 4) not following through instructions or failing to finish homework or work related tasks or chores, 5) Difficulty in organizing tasks and activities ending up being messy, 6) dislikes and avoids tasks that need sustained attention, 7) losing things, 8) easily distractible and 9) forgetful. I can see mothers of young boys reading this nodding their heads and wondering.

Majority of us would have one or more of these symptoms at some point and obviously not everyone can be diagnosed with ADHD. However, one can easily see how someone with a bias (a clinician, parent or the patient who has an intention to want the diagnosis) can easily convince themselves or others with a diagnosis of ADHD. Disruption or an impairment in day to day life is essential to diagnose the disorder, but even the impairment can be subjective: losing a key or forgetting appointments can bring a lot of distress and these are very common; anyone who looks at the lost and found bin in a middle school would know this well.

In the hyperactivity criteria, 6 out of the following 9 symptoms are required for a diagnosis: 1) fidgeting with hands, feet or squirming while sitting, 2) have difficulty sitting in one place for a sustained amount of time, 3) inappropriate running and climbing 4) not able to be quiet, 5) always being on the go, 6) talking excessively, 7) blurting out answers inappropriately, 8) difficulty waiting his or her turn, and 9) interrupting or intruding others.

Causes

Cause of ADHD is unknown. Like other mental illnesses, it also runs in the family and so believed to have a genetic basis. ADHD used to be known as minimal brain dysfunction or minimal brain damage, implying some insult to the brain and its development. Patients with mild intellectual disability have higher incidence of ADHD. Premature birth, low birth weight, brain injury from trauma or infection, neglect, abuse, exposure to chemicals like lead, seem to increase the incidence of ADHD. Similarly, prenatal exposure to drugs, alcohol, chemicals, or infectious agents lead to higher incidence of ADHD. There is no clear evidence for a high sugar diet, processed foods, or watching TV causing ADHD.

Sleep, or lack if it is an important aspect of a child or a teen with attentional problems. 95% of children with obstructive sleep apnea report attentional impairment. All of us know how cognitively impaired we would be if we do not sleep well. In obstructive sleep apnea (OSA), the airway is blocked in deep sleep, making the individual snore and choke, which in turn makes them "wake up" or go from deeper stages (3 or 4) to superficial stages of sleep. It is equivalent to waking up someone or prodding them several times in sleep (often dozens of times). 20% to 30% of children diagnosed with ADHD also seem to have OSA. ADHD may have associated problems with sleep, but a large number of children and teens are sleep deprived, or at least have poor sleep habits that might contribute to the attentional impairment. The modern lifestyle, with poor and inadequate sleep, late night screen time, alcohol at night, and coffee in the morning associated with a pressure or need to accomplish more than what we physically can, might lead us all to believe in ADHD and believe in the need for a boost[4].

Neurochemistry

ADHD seems to involve the dopaminergic system and adrenergic system. A reduction of dopamine is hypothesized to be associated with poor attention. Medications that increase dopamine seem to help ADHD.

Treatment

Most of us with suboptimal attention span learn to live with it. Our attention and focus increase when we are curious or when we do something important, interesting or enjoyable. So, as we grow older and choose the subjects and professions we like (who wants to study math after high school?), our attentional problem becomes more and more manageable (with a lot of coffee that is). In addition, at least half of the children with attentional problems seem to grow out of it, sooner or later. However, ADHD can be very disabling and disrupting for the child, family and the classroom. Management of ADHD is both psychosocial as well as psychopharmacological.

Psychosocial management includes psychoeducation, behavioral therapy, and support. A lot can be achieved by helping the kid get or-

---

4 Of all the diagnosis the author was given or considered, ADHD came under unusual circumstances. He was "diagnosed" by a colleague who insisted that he takes stimulants and see someone in therapy in a very inappropriate, unsolicited work setting. Annoyed by the violation of his personal space, he quipped; "if only I can find a reason for all my shortcomings, it would be nice." The unsolicited "consultant" did not seem to appreciate his sense of humor.

ganized and helping him to manage time. We all function better with structure, rules and consequences. No one wants to crash a car, and everyone knows how to be careful when we drive, but without traffic rules and traffic lights, I am sure we all would be behaving like ADHD kids. Time management tools like schedules, timetables, and reminders help along with simple rewards for better behavior, better sleep improve attention. Aerobic exercise like running or jogging in the morning seem to have a lot of positive effects for the brain, including improved mood, attention and problem-solving skills.

Many patients with mild to moderate attention problems can be managed without stimulants. A thorough investigation of contributing factors such as sleep, discipline and work habits should be conducted, and improved sleep habits and regular exercise would help a long way with our attentional capacity. Stimulants should be the last resort.

The mainstay of pharmacological treatment of ADHD or ADD is stimulants. All stimulants are related to amphetamine salts, and act in the same way. Stimulants are neurotoxic and have an addiction potential. The issue of addiction and stimulant use in ADHD is debatable. It is possible that kids with ADHD have a higher chance of developing addiction later in life, especially to stimulants. The issue of whether the treatment with stimulants increases the chance of addiction due to exposure or decrease the chance because the treatment keeps them away from drugs, is unresolved. In the same manner, it is unclear whether taking stimulants during crucial neurodevelopmental period helps or hurts, with its influence on the developing brain. However, severely ill patients with ADHD do benefit from them and it is important to remember that higher doses are harmful immediately, as well as in the long term. Stimulants should not be used routinely and should be reserved for severe cases. But, the attitude of the parent and clinician may influence this decision greatly. Stimulants stunt growth and it is a concern for premature babies who are behind in the growth chart. Stimulants of any kind can cause or exacerbate psychosis and it is unclear whether use of stimulants during development increases the chance of psychosis later on.

Medication	Dose	Halflife
Methylphenidate	5 to 60 mg	4-12 hours
Amphetamine	5 to 40 mg	9-11 hours

Medication	Dose	Halflife
Amphetamine/dextro-amphetamine	10 to 60 mg	4-12 hours
Dextroamphetamine	10 to 60 mg	12 hours
Dexmethylphenidate	10 to 60 mg	3-4 hours
Lisdexamfetamine	10 to 60 mg	3-5 hours
Nonstimulants		
Atomoxetine	10-100 mg	21.6 hours
Guanfacine	1 to 4 mg	17 hours

Non-stimulant medications used for ADHD include atomoxetine, guanfacine, clonidine and bupropion. Bupropion is actually a stimulant but is milder than the others and so has less addiction potential but less effective than the others. Atomoxetine is classified as a norepinephrine reuptake inhibitor, and it leads to an increase in norepinephrine in the brain. Guanfacine and clonidine are alpha adrenergic receptor agonists and are used to treat high blood pressure, ADHD, anxiety and drug withdrawal (clonidine). These are non-addictive and are proven to help. Antidepressants have also been shown to help children with attention deficit, with or without the presence of depression or anxiety.

Intellectual Disabilities (ID)

Previously referred to as mental retardation, this new terminology or euphemism, is preferred by DSM-5 because of the derogatory use of the term "mental retardation" or "retard." In fact, the term "mental retardation" itself was created to replace the then derogatory word "moron," which in turn was implemented to replace the derogatory "simpleton." Now, use of the term mental retardation is officially banned in US government documents. In 2010, president Barack Obama signed a law called "Rosa's Law" which bars the use of the term "mental retardation" or the word "retard" from government documents[5].

From early 20th century to early 21st century, the designation of the disability was based on the IQ score. As it sounds horrible now, the official classification of ID in early 20th century was, idiot with IQ less than 25, imbecile (25 to 50) and moron (50-70) which later corresponded to severe, moderate, and mild mental retardation. In addition to the change in nomenclature, the DSM 5 also moved from determining the

[5] Rosa Marcelino was a 9-year-old girl with Down's syndrome. She was deemed "mentally retarded" in her school. But her family did not want to accept the label and fought to take the word out officially. Rosa and her family (siblings Nick, 14 and Gigi,12) worked on the petition to help pass the law.

disorder with IQ score alone to impairment in three domains: conceptual, social and practical. Such a change moves the emphasis from intelligence to ability or disability, at least to a certain extent. DSM-5 also moved from the use of multiaxial diagnosis, where mental retardation used to be diagnosed in axis II.

Although ID have been recognized since ancient times, a formal measure of IQ or psychometry started only in the 20th century. In the early 1900s, the French government commissioned Alfred Binet to device a test of intelligence to help place children with disability. In 1916 it was adapted to the US population, and introduced as the Stanford-Binet test. Now, there are multiple tests for cognition and IQ. IQ testing is a controversial topic, and criticisms include a lack of cultural sensitivity, gender bias and bias against minorities. It is also criticized for not measuring creativity or emotional intelligence. Like in many mental illnesses, when the disability or impairment is severe, it is rather clear, and when it is in the borderline, it becomes confusing and debatable. An IQ score of 70 used to be the cut off for a designation of mental retardation, which, one can imagine may cause problems for those on the border especially when the assessment error itself can be plus or minus 3.

An individual's IQ is measured against the population average, which is determined at 100 with a standard deviation of 15. The scoring follows the normal distribution and the Bell curve: 68% would fall within one standard deviation of the mean (85 to 115) and 95% would fall between two standard deviations (70 and 130). The rest (5%) include 2.5% on each end of individuals with IQ above 130 and 2.5% with low IQ, below 70. Mathematically 99.7% would fall between three standard deviations (55-145). The test does not or cannot measure above 145 or below 55[6].

The test materials are standardized to the age, and the scores yield a "mental age" which is then divided by the chronological age and multiplied by 100. So, a 10-year-old testing at a mental age of 10-year-old

---

[6] One might come across a lot of mythical stuff in the internet. IQ is scored against the norm as a comparison but not as an absolute score. The "normal" of 100 is actually decided by testing a large group and making the average at 100. Extreme measures (Like above 140) become unclear and mathematically dubious. There are ways to test "super intelligent" and there are various projection techniques to "measure" or estimate someone's high IQ. You may hear that Einstein had an IQ of 200 and such. I am not sure whether Einstein sat for an IQ test but the scale itself goes only up to 145 and anything above is not statistically normalized. However, an IQ of 130 is more than enough for someone to have a successful life or career in any job. An IQ of 140 or above is considered genius and there would be at least one or two in every class of 100 with that IQ. Work ethics, opportunity, and plain luck go a long way than an IQ of "200." Similarly, there is no ranking based on IQ, meaning someone is ranked as the best or second best or top ten in the world in IQ, it must be meant as a joke. Also, Mozart and Picasso are geniuses by any measure, but they may or may not score high in the IQ test.

would have a score of 100. If the child scores at a mental age of 8, his IQ would be 80, which is below average, and if he scores at a mental age of 12 it would be 120, above average.

The DSM-5 requires three criteria to be met for the diagnosis of ID including A) deficit in intellectual function (reasoning, problem solving, planning, abstract thinking, judgment, academic learning, and learning from experience), B) deficits in adaptive functioning, leading to failure in attaining personal independence and social responsibility and C) onset of these deficits in the developmental period. The severity of the disability is scored as mild, moderate, severe and profound.

Criterion A is assessed by observation, clinical assessment and formal IQ testing. Criterion B emphasizes impairment in three areas: conceptual, social and practical. The conceptual domain includes skills in language, reading, writing, math, reasoning, knowledge and memory, the social domain includes empathy, social judgment, interpersonal communication skills, the ability to form and retain friendships, and similar social skills. The practical domain revolves around self-management such as personal care, money management, job, recreation, managing and maintaining living situation, and organizing work or school related tasks. The severity rating, mild, moderate, severe and profound are assessed using the above three domains. Individuals with severe disability frequently have physical abnormalities that impact functioning level. They may also have comorbid conditions such as ADHD, autism, seizures, anxiety or depression affecting the disability.

ID is frequently caused by chromosomal or genetic abnormalities (referred here as syndromal causes) such as Down's syndrome, fragile X syndrome and metabolic abnormalities such as phenylketonuria, but it can occur without any obvious physical or physiological causes. Preventable causes, such as hypothyroidism or infections, should be ruled out or treated appropriately. There is no pharmacological treatment for ID, but the comorbid conditions, if any, need to be treated accordingly. Behavioral problems, anger and agitation pose challenges in managing these patients. These individuals lack self-control and have less of a filter to control their behavior, especially when they are frustrated. Sedatives like lorazepam may be helpful in cases of agitation but these drugs can also disinhibit someone and make the behavior worse. Evidence for prevention or reduction of behavioral problems with medication is only anecdotal. Some benefit from stimulants that improve their learning and behavior. Lithium, valproate, carbamazepine, propranolol and naltrexone have been used to treat associated behavioral problems and agitation. Antipsychotics are also used often. SSRIs and buspirone are occasionally used for behavioral problems associated with anger and frustration.

Diagnosis of comorbid conditions such as depression or anxiety may be difficult because of the patient's disability. Depression and anxiety may present as agitation or anger. They can get psychosis but sometimes, individuals with ID are misdiagnosed as having psychosis and schizophrenia. For example, having an imaginary friend and talking to them may be seen as a delusion and hallucination[7]. Rituals and rocking behavior are often mistaken as OCD. Patients may have seizures or seizure like events (episodic behavioral disturbances, occasional confusion or loss of awareness). They may not have any EEG abnormalities but might benefit from the use of antiepileptics such as valproic acid or carbamazepine. It is prudent to have a meeting with the family or caregivers to explain the realistic expectation and implications of treatment options. It is important to explain to them that there is no proven treatment, and the treatment is for the symptoms. It is important to minimize side effects.

Motor Disorders

There are three developmental motor disorders described here: Developmental Coordination Disorder, Stereotypic Movement Disorder and Tic Disorders (in addition to the usual "other" and unspecified categories in the DSM).

Developmental Coordination Disorder

This condition is diagnosed when children do not acquire the motor coordination skills expected at the level of their age, and it significantly interferes with activities of daily living. This starts at the developmental age and is not explained by other disabilities such as intellectual disability, visual impairment or neuromuscular diseases.

Children may differ in the rate of acquiring fine motor skills and this is rarely diagnosed before age 5. They may appear clumsy and may have difficulty using tools or toys. This may become more apparent as they get older and are expected to do more and more demanding things from buttoning a shirt, tying the lace or playing in groups. It is estimated that 5 to 6% of children between ages 6 and 11 have this disorder. Although they improve as they get older, 50 to 70% continue to have problems. Like many neurodevelopmental disorders, it is common among children born prematurely or low-birth-weight children. Any

---

[7] A diagnosis of schizophrenia is debatable in patients with ID. Conceptually, any individual needs to have a fully formed ego functioning or logical thinking before they can develop schizophrenia. But ID patients can have psychosis. They are ideally diagnosed with psychosis not otherwise specified or psychosis secondary to a medical condition. However, treatment is the same.

prenatal exposure to alcohol, nicotine, drugs or infections also increase the probability. There is a high comorbidity with ADHD and other neurodevelopmental disorders.

Stereotypic Movement Disorder

Stereotypic movements are repetitive, apparently purposeless complex movements, like rocking back and forth, biting, head banging, rhythmic movement of hands, flicking fingers in front of the face, etc. These need to start during the developmental years, and interfere with personal, social and academic activities to constitute a disorder. They are different from tics and other neurological or psychiatric conditions (chorea, trichotillomania or OCD). Tics start late (4-6 years of age) and vary in presentation. Stereotypic movements start earlier, more complex but not as variable as tics and persist over time. These are common in patients with autism spectrum disorder, and intellectual disability and they may be diagnosed separately, if the behavior results in injury or discomfort.

Tic Disorders

Among the developmental motor disorders, tic disorders or Tourette' syndrome is the most popular or notorious in pop culture, partly because some kids with this disorder blurt out obscenities, which is not as common, but sensationalized in the popular media.

Tics are very common. A lot of us go through periods of time when we have some simple motor or vocal tics like eye blinking or throat clearing which are generally transient, frequently unnoticed and disappear without intervention. We may not even notice people with these tics and generally dismiss them as a habit. For a diagnosis of Tourette's syndrome an individual should have multiple motor tics and one or more phonic tics, that start before the age 18 and persist at least a year. If an individual has only motor or phonic tics, they are diagnosed with persistent motor (or phonic) tic disorder, and if they are present for less than a year, they are diagnosed provisionally.

Tics typically start between ages 4 and 6, reaching a peak around 11 or 12 years of age. They wax and wane over the years and get better as they become adults, although it may persist in severe form in some adults. Tics can involve any part of the body, from simple tics like clearing the throat or blinking the eyes, to complex with a series of jerky movements, or orchestrated and elaborate, yet purposeless rituals that involve the whole body. They can injure themselves by constant movements, or injure others by throwing, attacking or behaving recklessly. Patients and families may be too embarrassed to go out or to interact with others, affecting the individual at school, home, and social situations.

Patients recognize that the tics are purposeless and are able to control or stop them at times. Some feel an urge or a premonition preceding the tics and a relief or satisfaction after. Sometimes tics are precipitated by a stimulus - a sound, smell, vision or even a thought. Occasionally they repeat or copy what others do (echopraxia). The phonic tics can range from a simple cough, or a meaningless syllable (Ta, Ka), bird or animal noises, to complex words, or sentences, including obscene words or songs. They may repeat what they say over and over or repeat what others say (echolalia).

Nervousness, tiredness, stress, or excitement can worsen the tics. They also worsen when observed, due to the anxiety and embarrassment. The severity of the illness varies with the number of tics and how they interfere with the day to day functioning. At its worst, it can happen all the time and interfere everything in the kid's life to a point he or she may become isolated, lag behind in academics and have a low self-esteem and depression. There is a high comorbidity with ADHD, OCD, anxiety disorders and depression.

Treatment of tics is complex. There is no cure. Antipsychotics, typical and atypical are frequently used and are beneficial but, severe side effects discourage clinicians and parents from using these medications long term. Alpha adrenergic agonists clonidine and guanfacine are used with limited success. CBT is useful when there is a comorbid OCD. Psychoeducation, support and treatment of comorbid conditions are also helpful. Comprehensive Behavioral Intervention for Tics (CBIT) is a program that involves employing a competing response or doing something opposite of the tic (Habit Reversal Therapy) to mitigate the symptoms. There are some new medications in the pipeline including VMAT2 inhibitors such as deutetrabenazine in the testing phase.

Specific Learning Disorders

Learning disabilities are more common than we think, and about 10 to 15% of children are affected but, it seems many of them grow out of this, and the adult prevalence is estimated only at 4%. It is two to three times more common in males than females. The cause is unknown, but they run in the families suggesting a genetic basis. They are common, like many developmental disorders, among babies born prematurely, or children who had some insult to the brain during developmental years. Difficulties in acquiring academic skills or learning disorders do not mean that the individual is developmentally delayed or less capable than others. Some extremely successful people including, a Nobel Prize winning scientist have dyslexia[8].

Academic skills are taught and acquired as the child starts going to school in contrast to developmental milestones. So, these disorders usually become apparent as the child goes to school. However, preschool children show some struggle to use words or sounds. They would show disinterest or frustration when they are involved in plays that include rhyming or words and songs. They may continue to have "baby talk" longer than their peers. But their difficulties become apparent when they start school. Some children catch up and improve as they get older, but learning disorders are usually lifelong. The symptoms vary in presentation depending upon the severity, coping skills, comorbidity and the intellectual ability.

The DSM-5 diagnostic category lists 6 specific learning difficulties in the areas of 1) reading and sounding out words 2) reading to understand (comprehension), 3) spelling, 4) writing, 5) mathematics and use of numbers, and 6) mathematical reasoning. The affected children must be substantially and quantifiably below the level of their peers and the difficulties must interfere with occupational performance or daily activities. They are unrelated to intellectual disabilities and should be apparent in school age. The diagnosis also requires specifiers in reading (word reading accuracy, reading rate or fluency, reading comprehension), in writing (spelling accuracy, grammar and punctuation accuracy, clarity and accuracy of written expression), and in math (number sense, memorization of arithmetic facts, accurate or fluent calculation and accurate math reasoning).

While learning disorders can be disabling and may interfere with day to day living, a number of other factors such as choice of career, level of general intelligence, support, coping skills, and even the environment can influence the success and wellbeing of the individual.

Communication Disorders

These include, speech sound disorder (articulation or creating appropriate sounds), childhood-onset fluency disorder (Stuttering), language disorder and social (Pragmatic) communication disorder.

Speech Sound Disorder

Until age three, children shorten words and syllables as they learn to speak, and until age seven, they may not fully master complex sounds required for normal speech. The sounds in speech development are di-

[8] Dr. Carol Greider is one of the three winners of Nobel Prize for medicine in 2009. She had difficulty in reading, writing and even speaking but found ways to cope with the disability. She says that the determination and her will to overcome the disability helped her accomplish more.

vided as early 8s, middle 8s and late 8s[9]. Children with speech sound disorder have difficulties in late 8s ("sh" as in "sheep", /s/ as in "see", "th" as in "think", "th" as in "that", /r/ as in "red", /z/ as in "zoo", /l/ as in "like", and "zh" as in "measure"). Speech sound disorder is a persistent difficulty in speech sound production, which makes verbal communication difficult, as some of the spoken words or sounds become difficult to understand, interfering with day to day activities. The symptoms should start early and may not be explained by neuromuscular abnormalities such as cleft palate or cerebral palsy. It seems that these children lack the ability to fully understand the sound of speech and have difficulty in mastering the coordination of muscles to produce the accurate sound. This condition may be variable depending upon the deficit and the children improve as they grow older, or when they engage in speech therapy.

Childhood-Onset Fluency Disorder (Stuttering)

Stuttering is a disturbance in the normal fluency of speech in which one of the following: 1) sound or syllable repetition (ca ca ca cat,), 2) prolongation of sounds (Ca-aaaw-t), 3) pauses within a word, 4) pauses in the speech that may be silent or with a sound, 5) circumlocutions (substituting words to avoid problematic words), 6) producing words with excessive tension, and 7) repetition of monosyllabic words (I-I-I-I like cat). Individuals with stuttering have anxiety about speaking and their communication is affected.

Stuttering is prevalent in about 1% of the population. The cause is unknown, but it runs in families, suggesting a genetic influence. It is more common in boys than girls (3:1) and generally starts around 2 to 7 years of age. They start with occasional repetitions that worsen over time. As they grow older, they develop coping skills, by avoiding speaking in public, or limiting themselves to monosyllabic conversation. Anxiety and fear of embarrassment may limit their social activities, and it can be crippling in teen years. However, it is estimated that 65% to 85% of children grow out of it before they reach adulthood.

The treatment of stuttering is behavioral. Stuttering may not be a behavioral or learned problem but there is a significant associated anxiety which worsens the stuttering. A simple acknowledgment of stuttering by the stutterer and a non-judgmental audience reduce the stuttering. The kids are taught to speak slowly, with a gentle or easy onset

---
9 Early 8 - /m/ as in "mama", /b/ as in "baby", Y as in "you", /n/ as in "no", /w/ as in "we", /d/ as in "daddy", /p/ as in "pop" and /h/ as in "hi".
Middle 8: /t/ as in "two", "ng" as in running, /k/ as in "cup", /g/ as in "go", /f/ as in "fish", /v/ as in "van", "ch" as in "chew" and "j" as in "jump".
Late 8: "sh" as in "sheep", /s/ as in "see", "th" as in "think", "th" as in "that", /r/ as in "red", /z/ as in "zoo", /l/ as in "like", and "zh" as in "measure".

of voicing, smooth transition of words and with a sing song prosody[10]. Interestingly, stutterers do not stutter when they sing. CBT focused on anxiety reduction is helpful.

Language Disorder

Language Disorder consists deficits in comprehension (receptive) or production (expressive) of language. Affected children do not acquire adequate vocabulary, do not learn to master sentence structure, and have impairments in the ability to have a meaningful conversation. These language disabilities lead to functional limitation, start in the early developmental period and are not accountable by other neuromuscular problems.

These children learn new words later than their peers, have very limited vocabulary and struggle with grammar. They have difficulty in understanding instructions, narrating events and engaging in a conversation. Although some improve, the deficits remain through life. Hearing difficulties, neurological and intellectual disabilities should be considered while treating these patients. Behavioral intervention with reinforcement for learning and mastering language, and additional coaching are needed for management.

Social (Pragmatic) Communication Disorder

This disorder is characterized by difficulties in the use of verbal and nonverbal communication in a social setting: greeting or sharing information appropriately, ability to change the manner of communication for the context (school vs. family vs peer or an adult), ability to maintain the basic etiquette of a social conversation, including taking turns or rephrasing appropriately and understanding implicit or hidden meanings (idioms, innuendo, metaphor or even context dependent use of words). These deficits start during the developmental period, impair or interfere with functioning and are not attributed to neuropsychological causes like autism or an intellectual disability. The treatment involves training and coaching. Some get better as they grow older and develop compensatory mechanisms, but symptoms may stay for life.

Elimination Disorders (Enuresis and Encopresis)

DSM-5 lists enuresis (passing urine in inappropriate places) and encopresis (passing of feces in inappropriate places) as two disorders. Babies obtain bladder and bowel control by age 1-3, rarely beyond 4 for bowel and 5 for bladder control and so enuresis is diagnosed after age 5 and encopresis after age 4. The training and mastery of bladder and

---

10 Marilyn Monroe had stuttering and to suppress or avoid stuttering she learned to speak in a sing song manner which accentuated her image and appeal.

bowel control are influenced by a number of factors including child's intellectual capacity, social maturity, cultural and psychological factors.

Enuresis

Bed wetting is more common among boys than girls. It can be nocturnal or diurnal. For a diagnosis, the child needs to void urine in inappropriate places at least twice weekly for three months, and they should be at least 5-year-old. Micturition is a complex neuromuscular event that involves the central, peripheral, and autonomic nervous system, including motor, sensory and reflex neurons. In infants, when the bladder becomes full it makes the detrusor muscle contract "automatically" and they void. As they grow, they develop better sensation of fullness, motor control of the bladder, and master their "need to go." 82% of 2-year-olds, have this problem and by the time they are 5, only 5-10% have it and less than 1% of adolescents experience this. Although this happens more at night and in sleep, it can also happen during the daytime. There is no relationship to sleep, its stages or sleep problems. Rarely, a child may do this intentionally to gain attention.

Some children may produce excessive amount of urine due to fluid intake or low secretion of antidiuretic hormone, which normally increases in sleep. Typically, children with enuresis reach full bladder and empty it in bed. If they void little by little instead of emptying, it may reflect an organic problem like urinary tract infection or neuromuscular abnormality. Enuresis runs in families supporting a genetic basis, but sociocultural factors, and attitude of the parents may also play a role. A gradual improvement with age and spontaneous remission is common.

Frequently, a better toilet training is adequate to address the problem. These include; training the child to hold for longer periods of time (to improve holding capacity), learn to understand when it is too long (fullness and pain), regular bathroom visits, fluid restriction before sleep, and emptying before bedtime or earlier in the night. Most of the kids benefit with simple behavioral intervention - especially fluid restriction and voiding before bedtime. A diary, or record of voiding, kept visibly in the child's room along with a star chart for good behavior goes a long way in assessing the problem as well as treating it.

Medications are rarely used and only in intractable cases. Desmopressin is an analogue of vasopressin, or antidiuretic hormone, taken before bedtime as a wafer or nasal spray will greatly reduce the urine output. Tricyclic antidepressants have also been used with good success, but they have serious side effects of dry mouth and constipation, and so should be used sparingly. Medication treatment should be combined with behavioral intervention and training. Emotional and interpersonal issues, especially self-esteem issues, should be addressed. The Bell-and-pad method is a kind of behavioral intervention. The child wears a battery-operated fluid sensor in the underwear or on a mat on the bed, that activates a loud alarm when it gets wet waking the child up and interrupting the voiding. This is supposed to "train" the child to avoid bed wetting but is rarely used.

Encopresis

Encopresis is passing feces in inappropriate places and times. For a diagnosis, this needs to happen at least once a month for three months and cause psychological distress and interference in day to day life. This can be involuntary or voluntary. Voluntary behavior may result from the child's attempt to get negative attention from parents or caregivers, or regressive behavior upon the birth of a younger sibling. Involuntary encopresis may happen because the child is preoccupied with something else or has poor sphincter control, or from chronic constipation and overflow. 90 percent of encopresis result from the interplay of behavioral and physiological factors. The child may habitually hold feces for long periods of time, leading to constipation, impaction and overflow that gets out of his or her control. The constipation and impaction make defecation painful, leading the kid to hold more and thus worsening the condition. It is more common in boys than girls. Physiological causes including neuromuscular problems need to be ruled out. The treatment involves laxatives or stool softener for constipation and building discipline in toilet habits. Encopresis causes emotional and interpersonal conflicts in the family and self-esteem issues for the child. Reassurance and support may be required.

Disruptive, Impulse-control, and Conduct Disorders

Oppositional Defiant Disorder

> *"When my child was born, I thought, 'I never imagined I could feel this much love' and when she grew older, I thought 'I never imagined I could get this angry.'" - a loving mother...*

Parents of young children would vouch for this. Even the best-behaved children can be oppositional at times, and exhibit behaviors described here. I am sure, as children, we all would have pushed our parents to the edge at some point or other with our oppositional behavior. The DSM includes 8 symptoms of ODD in three categories including; angry/irritable mood (1-losing temper often, 2-easily annoyed, and angry, and 3 -being resentful), defiant behavior (4-arguing with adults or authority figures, 5-defying or refusing to comply with rules, 6-deliberately annoying others and 7-blaming others for their mistakes) and vindictiveness (8-being spiteful or vindictive - at least twice in the past 6 months).

It is not unusual for many children to exhibit these behaviors at some point, but a child with ODD is essentially defined by this kind of behavior. Their behavior would be extreme, consistent and constant to a point, that it can cause an extraordinary amount of frustration for the family, friends and school. This has to last for 6 months or more for a diagnosis. These behaviors typically start in preschool and are more common in boys at this age, but girls catch up around puberty. ODD is found to be prevalent in about 3% of children. Families may have different levels of tolerance that may enable or limit such behavior in children. Children with ADHD, depression, anxiety or other comorbid diagnoses may exhibit defiant behavior at times. Children with ODD with predominant symptoms of anger and irritability seem to have higher incidence of mood disorders later in life (and so, may benefit from antidepressants) and others who may have predominant defiance and behavioral problems are more prone for conduct disorder or personality disorders. Treatment involves training the child to develop anger management, impulse control and problem-solving ability. The family should also be involved in the counseling to identify behaviors that may enable the child's opposition.

Disruptive Mood Dysregulation Disorder

This is a similar condition to ODD in which the child is excessively irritable and angry, with frequent temper tantrums. This starts before age 10 but not diagnosed before age 6 or after age 18. These children are often diagnosed with bipolar disorder in childhood with an assumption that they would eventually develop mania, but they do not seem to. These children seem to develop anxiety disorders or mood disorders more so than bipolar as they grow older. The treatment may include stimulants, antidepressants and antipsychotics. Some clinicians use antiepileptic mood stabilizers like carbamazepine or oxcarbazepine or beta blockers like propranolol with variable success. Parental training and behavioral therapy for the child may help.

Intermittent Explosive Disorder

More common in boys, this disorder is characterized by a lack of control of aggressive impulses. They exhibit impulsive verbal or physical aggression towards others, animals or property (2-3 times a week for 3 months) or three episodes of physical aggression that results in property damage or injury in one year. Treatment with SSRIs, mood stabilizers (Oxcarbazepine, Carbamazepine, lithium) beta blockers (propranolol) and atypical antipsychotics (risperidone) have been shown to help these children. But the evidence is anecdotal.

Conduct Disorder

Conduct disorder is essentially antisocial personality disorder in adolescents. It is found to be prevalent at 9.5% (boys 12% and girls 7.5%) and of these, 40% of boys and 25% of girls eventually meet the criteria for antisocial personality disorder. It is believed that there is a subgroup of children who develop this before age 10, and they seem to have lasting behavioral problems, compared to those who develop this behavior as teens. Conduct disorder runs in families supporting a genetic etiology. However, parenting, household environment, sociocultural influences, and peer pressure contribute to the development of antisocial behavior.

Children with conduct disorder lack empathy or fear. They are bullies who initiate fights, use weapons, confront and steal, force others for sex and are cruel to others or animals. They may destroy property, set fires for fun or disobey age appropriate rules like staying out late, running away from home and being truant. They may also have associated illnesses including ADHD, learning difficulties, substance use, and ODD. Many of these children end up in juvenile justice system.

Kleptomania

Children or adults with Kleptomania have an uncontrollable impulse to steal something that may not have any value or importance to them. They have an urge to steal, which builds up, and only relieved with the theft. They frequently steal something trivial or that holds no value but important to the victim, like keys or photographs. It appears that people with kleptomania enjoy the panic and reaction of the victims. After stealing, they would join the victim searching for the lost item, offering words of support while misleading the victim at the same time. They seem to enjoy the victim's panic and their role as a savior. A good example is stealing textbooks before exam and then helping the victim with personal notes. The psychopathology of kleptomania seems to be related to obsessive compulsive disorder or addiction. SSRIs, mood stabilizers, and opioid antagonists (reduces craving in addicts) are found to be useful along with behavioral therapy.

Pyromania

It is a primal instinct to start or watch fires, which can be calming. However, individuals with pyromania have a strong urge to start fires, with no motivation other than the relief of the pressure from the impulse. There is no other motivation than the fire itself. Similar to kleptomania, some individuals may start fire and help the firefighters.

Compulsive Shopping

Compulsive shopping or compulsive buying disorder is also driven by an impulse that leads to pleasure or relief when completed. Patients enjoy the act of buying and become indiscriminate to a point they hurt their finances and personal life. They also resemble OCD or addiction and the treatment is similar to behavioral therapy, group therapy, support or SSRIs.

Internet Addiction

There is a lot written and discussed about "Internet Addiction" on the internet. While it is debated whether this is a bona fide disease or not, a behavior that leads to impairment in the day to day life is a problem. The treatment involves education on time management and discipline. Comorbid conditions need to be evaluated.

Video Game Addiction

This seems to be more valid than the internet addiction. While video gaming, or at times referred as "gaming" can follow the same path or mechanism of addition including intense preoccupation about the next fix, spending an inordinate amount of time, money and effort on gaming to a point the child or adult compromises on his (or her) life's goals. Treatment approach is similar to addiction.

Chapter 15

Sleep Disorders

Normal Sleep

We spend about a third of our lives sleeping. Sleep is believed to stabilize and restore the brain and body for optimal neurobehavioral functioning in the following day. While the inherent biological need for sleep is felt by everyone, the fact that we evolved with such a need is a scientific enigma, because sleep is not safe - in the evolutionary, predatory context. A sleeping organism is defenseless and vulnerable. Mammals, reptiles, amphibians, fish and even simpler worms and insects sleep or have the need to sleep. Dolphins and whales, who need to come to the surface to breathe, sleep with one half of their brain awake and the corresponding eye open. They even swim in circles with the open eye looking outside. Apparently, the natural selection comes from the advantages sleep brings to the wakefulness. Sleep is essential for life, and people can die from lack of sleep[1].

On average, healthy adults need about 7.5 to 8.5 hours of sleep every day. Sleep, along with the blissfully altered consciousness, that is turned on and off - who knows how - is a peaceful state of mind and body during which time we do not respond to external stimuli, ignore sensory input, and lose control over our muscles. And, we recover all these upon waking up. Sleep is a major homeostatic biological function with specific characteristics: it is controlled by a circadian rhythm - a biological clock that runs in cycles of about 24 hours[2] - to maintain the

---

1 There is a condition known as Fatal Familial Insomnia, an autosomal dominant disorder with a mutation of the protein PrPC. The illness manifests in the 50s when the patient becomes progressively unable to sleep, develop multitude of psychiatric symptoms from anxiety, psychosis to dementia before dying in a year or two.
2 Circadian rhythm is maintained by suprachiasmatic nucleus whose neurons fire in synchrony to maintain the roughly 24-hour cycle with the help of external sources of time known as Zeitgebers (time givers in German).

sleep wake cycle. Its intensity and duration are affected by the homeostatic need (or how tired one feels). The whole body, even at the cellular or system level slows down or goes to sleep at the cellular level. Sleep has a complex architecture with several overlapping stages as described below.

Sleep is divided as non-Rapid Eye Movement (NREM) sleep and Rapid Eye Movement sleep (REM) - the part of sleep when eyeballs dart sideways, which can be observed underneath the closed eyelids. We sleep in cycles that last about 90 (80-120) minutes, and each cycle starts with NREM sleep, which goes through stages 1-4 before entering REM sleep. We complete about 3 to 6 cycles a night. The cycles vary as the night goes on, and the proportion of REM sleep increases from 10% in the first cycle to 20 to 25% later on. We dream during the REM sleep.

NREM Sleep

NREM Stage 1 (5%) is the transition from wakefulness to sleep. EEG shows low amplitude alpha waves with a frequency of 8-13 Hz (cycles per second). When we are awake, we have beta (12-30hz and gamma 25-100 Hz). Stage 2 (45%) is the bulk of the sleep accounting for 45%-50% of total sleep hours, in which, alpha waves give way to slower theta waves (4-7 Hz) on EEG. A couple of interesting EEG phenomenon occur during this time called K-complexes and sleep spindles. K-complexes are sudden, sharp, high-voltage negative waves on EEG believed to occur as a response to internal stimuli because the same waves can be observed while awake in response to external stimuli like loud sound. Sleep spindles are low voltage, high frequency waveforms on EEG that look like a spindle. Sleep spindles are believed to represent consolidation of memory and learning. Stage 3 (25% with stage 4) is called slow wave sleep or deep sleep because the EEG is dominated by slow delta waves (1-2 Hz). Stage 4 consists of delta waves. Stages 3 and 4 are called deep sleep and if woken up at this stage, people have a difficult time to recover and feel groggy for some time. During NREM sleep, the brain and body seem to rest. Body temperature falls, breathing becomes uniform and regular, heart rate is slower and regular, and the kidneys produce less urine. But, some functions like digestion, cell repair and growth - with an increase in the secretion of growth hormone - happen during this time. It seems that the body physiologically reboots and retools itself on a daily basis, that helps us live longer; more or less like servicing our car.

REM Sleep

REM sleep (25%) has alpha waves but it is different from the rest of the sleep by the presence of rapid eye movements and a complex behavior of the brain and body. REM sleep is also called paradoxical sleep, or desynchronized sleep, because the physiological state and EEG resemble wakefulness. In addition to dreaming actively, during REM sleep, the heart rate, arterial pressure, and breathing become irregular. The brain seems to cease control of these functions during this time. In addition, internal temperature regulation stops in this stage, making the body vulnerable to the temperature of the surrounding, the reason why we feel cold (or hot) and curl up and get under sheets to reduce heat loss. The muscles lose tone and erection of penis or engorgement of clitoris occurs. The jerky eye movements are visible for the observer, and some act out the dreams (fight, smile, defend or respond). REM sleep is strange!

Sleep is probably the single most important objective/measurable physiological function in mental health, and every patient should be asked about sleep in every visit. The relationship of sleep to mental illness is bidirectional - poor sleep can precipitate, cause or worsen mental illnesses, it can be a symptom or sign of illness or severity of the illness. Sleep is impaired in depression, anxiety, PTSD, schizophrenia, mania and others. Almost all mental illnesses and substance use can impact sleep adversely. A lack of sleep can worsen or precipitate relapse in psychosis and mania. Insomnia is common in depression, and patients with both insomnia and depression do not do well. Interestingly, sleep deprivation (not inadequate sleep) seems to help with depression. Sleep problems are prominent in anxiety disorders. Panic attacks can occur in sleep. PTSD symptoms such as nightmares interfere with sleep. Poor sleep worsens the symptoms and when sleep is improved, the patient feels much better even if the symptoms take time to resolve.

Psychiatric medications, with or without sedation as a side effect can influence sleep. Norepinephrine and serotonin suppress REM sleep and acetylcholine initiates REM sleep. Antidepressants that increase norepinephrine and serotonin, as well as anticholinergic action of tricyclics can suppress REM. Antipsychotics with histamine blocking properties can cause sedation. Norepinephrine controls production and release of melatonin which enables sleep and dopamine blocks the effects of norepinephrine. Considering the complex interaction of sleep and mental illness, it is important that we evaluate sleep and the factors that affect sleep (stress, sleep habits, obesity and sleeping environment, drug and alcohol use etc.).

Sleep Hygiene

Good sleep is essential for the homeostasis of the brain. Like many things, our body can be trained to get good quality natural sleep - with some discipline. The following are tips to improve sleep and sleep habits.

- Go to bed and wake up at the same time every day. This is very true the day after a bad night's sleep - like on weekends. In those days, even if you go to bed late, try not to sleep in, wake up at the same time and although the day may feel weary, wait it out until the bedtime next night for a better night's sleep. The irregular sleep schedule or habit is a major problem for many, young and old, and regularizing sleep habit might solve a lot of problems for the day.
- Do not use stimulants like caffeine or nicotine before sleep. In general caffeine should be avoided for about 8 hours before bedtime. Alcohol is a downer, but it still it interferes with sleep making it unsatisfactory. All psychoactive drugs should be avoided - preferably.
- Make the bedroom conducive for sleep: a quiet, cool (60-70oF), dark place is important. Recent research supports that the cool temperature is more important than darkness for a good night's sleep.
- Pre-sleep routine should be soothing and relaxing (reading a book). Avoid exercise or arguments before sleep. Screen time interferes with the body's ability to relax and should be kept at minimum.
- Try not to force sleep and only sleep when you are tired. If you cannot fall asleep in 20 minutes after going to bed or wake up in the middle of the night and cannot fall back to sleep in 20 minutes, consider some quiet activity like reading. Having the lights on can interfere with the internal clock. Natural light blocks the secretion of melatonin which coincides with waking up. Small, light, and early dinner with adequate fluids will decrease the chance of indigestion and thirst that can interfere with sleep.
- Aerobic exercise in the morning like running or jogging promotes good sleep at night. Exercise before sleep makes it difficult to fall asleep.
- Short naps, early in the afternoon should be avoided for a good night's sleep. However, siesta or a short nap in the afternoon is considered good for health, but it should be a regular habit[3].

---

3 Naps are said to reduce cardiac risk, increase memory and creativity. A 20-minute nap is more refreshing than a jolt of espresso, but it does not come in a handy disposable cup.

Sleep Disorders

Insomnia Disorder or sometimes known as "primary insomnia" is characterized by a dissatisfaction of sleep quality or quantity. About an astounding 30% of the population report poor sleep. The incidence is lower when stringent criteria like the DSM or polysomnography evidence are used, but it is amazing that so many people would complain about poor sleep. Poor sleep significantly affects quality of life, leading to less productive days, poor emotional and physical performance, and increases the chance of accidents.

Patients with insomnia have difficulty initiating or maintaining sleep. They may wake up randomly and find it difficult to fall back asleep. For a diagnosis, this should happen for three nights a week for three months, in spite of having adequate time for sleep (a lot of the 30% who complain about poor sleep may not have enough time allotted for sleep). The other requirements are - interference with day to day life, and exclusionary criteria of other sleep disorders, mental or physical illnesses. Temporary sleep problems may occur under stress, but they may not warrant medical attention.

Poor sleep, even for a few days, can cause bad mood, anxiety and irritability, and it is probably the most heard complaint from patients in a psychiatrist's office. The main feature of primary insomnia is hyperarousal. These patients have an inability to relax. They have hyperactive autonomic nervous system causing increased heart rate and blood pressure, elevated stress hormones such as cortisol, increased metabolism of the body and brain, with a high frequency beta activity in the EEG. They have longer sleep latency (time taken to fall asleep). Sleep studies are rarely done for insomnia unless some other problem is suspected, and the diagnosis is essentially clinical.

CBT for insomnia (CBTi)

Behavioral therapies for sleep and pain are becoming popular and are even reported to be superior to medications. The excessive use of controlled substances (in the USA), their addiction potential, and side effects are driving the field to look for safer alternatives. Insomnia, when it is chronic is almost always associated with poor sleep hygiene and poor sleep related behavior, which provides a window for behavioral intervention. For example, people with poor sleep tend to use excessive caffeine during the wakeful hours, which, in turn, interferes with sleep. CBTi includes weekly sessions for 6-8 weeks covering education about sleep hygiene, relaxation techniques, managing caffeine, alcohol and drug use. The cognitive restructuring technique includes sleep restriction and stimulus control.

Sleep restriction is a concept that restricts one to go to bed only to sleep[4]. The patients start a sleep diary that includes all information about sleep and caffeine, alcohol or drug use. The diary is used to direct the patient to go to bed only for the amount of time they actually sleep. They are not allowed to stay in bed longer than 20 minutes without sleeping, even if they feel tired. As the restriction is implemented, they will "train" themselves to sleep when they go to bed, and go to bed only when they are ready to sleep or about to fall asleep. As the association of sleep and the bed becomes stronger, they will gain confidence in their ability to fall asleep and lose their anxiety over sleep.

The goal is to train one's body to fall asleep when they want to, by going to bed when they are ready to fall asleep and by not going to bed when they are not ready to sleep. The stimulus control of CBTi is more or less the same as the sleep restriction. Here, the patient may have so much anxiety over sleep, the idea of going to bed or trying to fall asleep itself is anxiety provoking. Sleep restriction will "uncouple" this anxiety and train the body and mind to fall asleep as they hit the bed. Avoiding naps at random times, even when the patient is tired is also important in sleep restriction therapy. CBTi should be used with the practice of good sleep hygiene.

Practicing good sleep hygiene helps most patients. Over the counter, non-prescription drugs are recommended as first line of treatment. Melatonin (3 to 10 mg), (role of melatonin as a sleep inducer is questionable but placebo or not, it seems to help a lot of patients). Antihistamines, including diphenhydramine (25 to 50mg), doxylamine (10-50mg), chlorpheniramine (25-50mg) work well for sleep. Sedating antidepressants such as, trazodone 50 to 200 mg, doxepin 25 or 50 mg, and occasionally tricyclics like imipramine (25 mg to 50 mg) help with sleep. Hydroxyzine (25-50 mg), an antihistamine with anxiolytic properties is also used often. These have minimal addiction potential. Prescription drugs include benzodiazepines, benzodiazepine receptor agonists, gabapentin and others (table). Barbiturates were used in the past for sleep, but not anymore due to the addiction potential. Addiction potential should be part of the decision-making process when using these drugs.

Drug	Dose in mg	Half life
Benzodiazepines		
1. Estazolam (Prosom)	1-2	10-24
2. Flurazepam (Dalmane)	15-30	47-100
3. Quazepam (Doral)	7.5-25	25-84
4. Temazepam (Restoril)	7.5-30	4-18
5. Triazolam (Halcion)	0.125	2-3
6. Estazolam (Prosom)	0.25	8-13
Benzodiazepine receptor agonists		
1. Eszopiclone (Lunesta)	1-3	5-6
2. Zaleplon (sonata)	5-10	1-2
3. Zolpidem (Ambien)	5-10	2-3
4. Zolpidem ER	6.25-12.5	2-3
5. Zolpidem SL	1.75-3.5	2-3
Melatonin agonist		
1. Ramelteon	8	0.8-2
Orexin Antagonist		
1. Suvorexant	5-20	12

Hypersomnolence Disorder

Hypersomnolence disorder is characterized by excessive sleepiness despite sleeping well (at least 7 hours) the previous night. Sleepiness during daytime, need or urge for naps, long sleep periods (more than 9 hours), and difficulty waking up or feeling drowsy after waking up, are symptoms of hypersomnolence disorder. This should happen 3 times a week for 3 months and interfere with day to day work for a diagnosis. Other sleep disorders, mental or physical illness or drug use are excluded. This is generally a diagnosis of exclusion, but Multiple Sleep Latency Test is diagnostic (subject is allowed 20-minute naps five times with two-hour intervals in a daytime or wakeful period. The subject would fall asleep within 5 minutes on average showing that he or she is not able to stay awake or falls asleep easily). Associated conditions that may cause excessive sleepiness (narcolepsy or sleep apnea) must be identified and treated appropriately. Some individuals may have poor sleep hygiene and become extremely sleepy during working hours. They must be retrained to get regular sleep. Treatment of this condition includes psychostimulants such as modafinil or methylphenidate.

Narcolepsy

Narcolepsy is characterized by sudden uncontrollable urges to sleep leading to 10 to 20-minute naps, known as sleep attacks. The patients have excessive daytime sleepiness, cataplexy, sleep paralysis, hypnagogic and hypnopompic hallucinations, and inappropriate REM sleep. They get REM sleep within 10 minutes of sleep and the sleep attack can happen anytime under any circumstances (talking, driving, eating and even during sex). It is not an epilepsy or migraine. There seems to be a problem with the REM induction, and it seems to be related to a molecule called hypocretin.

Cataplexy

Cataplexy is a sudden loss of muscle tone for parts of the body, or entire body, making one fall without falling asleep. Strong emotions like laughter, anger or crying can precipitate cataplexy. Antidepressants including tricyclics, or SSRIs, are used with some success when there is cataplexy.

Sleep paralysis is a condition in which the mind is awake, but the body is not, that can happen in otherwise normal people while waking up.

Hypnagogic hallucination is a hallucination that happens when one tries to fall asleep and hypnopompic hallucinations occur during awakening. They are vivid, and last for a few seconds to few minutes. The patient is aware that these are unusual experiences and are not dreamlike. The patient may be half asleep and when they wake up, they immediately realize that it is not a dream and it is a "real" experience. These can happen in otherwise normal people, especially under stress. These are also common in people with other sleep disorders and epilepsy. The treatment of narcolepsy is with stimulants. Modafinil is a stimulant approved for narcolepsy and has fewer side effects than other conventional stimulants. Suppression of REM with antidepressants like SSRIs or tricyclics may help. Sleep hygiene and scheduled naps also help.

Sleep Apnea

Breathing-related sleep disorders include Obstructive Sleep Apnea (OSA), Central Sleep Apnea and Mixed Sleep Apnea. Sleep apnea is a common disease and the incidence has increased in the USA most likely due to the obesity epidemic.

Obstructive Sleep Apnea (OSA)

OSA is characterized by repetitive occurrence of brief episodes of obstruction of airways during sleep. It is common in men, obese and those who have a narrow airway due to small jaw (micrognathia), retracted jaw (retrognathia), large neck, or other nasopharyngeal abnormalities such as enlarged tonsils. Smoking, nasal congestion, alcohol and sedatives exacerbate or cause OSA.

When we sleep, the pharyngeal muscles relax, and tongue falls back, narrowing the airway. Among the obese, or those who already have a narrow pathway, the airway gets fully obstructed leading to choking, gasping, awakening or partial awakening in sleep. When this happens for 10 seconds it is called apnea, and when this is shorter or happens partially, it is known as hypopnea. The awakening is called respiratory effort related arousal (RERA). The severity of OSA is measured by the number of apneas, hypopneas and RERAs. Apneas are common in REM sleep but can occur in NREM 1 and NREM 2. Blood oxygen level goes down with apneas leading to further complications. Heavy snoring happens when the obstruction is partial.

Unrefreshing sleep at night, excessive daytime sleepiness, dry mouth, headache, irritability, heavy snoring, along with the above risk factors, should raise the suspicion for OSA. Choking in sleep, or sudden awakening with a feeling of choking, may be a telltale sign of OSA. OSA can lead to hypertension, weight gain, cardiac arrhythmias, stroke, fatigue and complications with anesthesia - and a sleep deprived partner due to the snoring.

Typically, patients are diagnosed with a polysomnography where they measure the sleep architecture with EEG, blood oxygenation level, heart rate, and video monitoring of sleep. There is a home diagnosis kit available now. The treatment for OSA involves using a small machine that blows air into the airway overcoming the resistance. Continuous Positive Airway Pressure (CPAP) is most commonly used. Some people who have difficulty exhaling against pressure are prescribed a Bilevel Positive Airway Pressure (BPAP) machine. There are newer machines that automatically adjust the pressure depending upon the need (APAP). The CPAP and BPAP need to be calibrated after the sleep study, which is either done on a different night or the same night (known as split study). Some people with narrow airways may benefit from surgery or custom-made retractors. Mild apneas can be managed with oral appliances or mouthguards made to stop snoring. Sleeping on the side reduces the blockage of airways and some patients are recommended to secure a tennis ball in the back, which will prevent them from sleeping on the back (might wake them up anyways as they roll). No medication is seen beneficial but tricyclics that reduce REM may reduce the apneas.

Central Sleep Apnea is a rare condition in which the central nervous system may fail to initiate breathing. As opposed to OSA, patients are not seen to have respiratory effort, which is seen with choking in OSA.

Circadian Rhythm Sleep Disorders

Circadian (Latin for "about a day") rhythm makes several bodily functions cycle in 24 hours. The suprachiasmatic nucleus in hypothalamus (just above the optic chiasm), that fires independently in a 24-hour cycle, is the pacemaker for the circadian rhythm. The timely firing of the suprachiasmatic nucleus is inherent, but the body also takes cues from things like daylight (Zeitgebers, or time givers in German) to reset the body to time changes, like in intercontinental travel. Besides sleep wake cycle, melatonin level, cortisol secretion and core body temperature are influenced by the circadian rhythm.

The DSM-5 lists 6 disorders; 1) Delayed Sleep Phase type - people feel fresh in the evening and stay up late (night owls), 2) Advanced Sleep Phase Type – people who sleep early and wake up early, 3) Irregular Sleep-Wake Type where the sleep wake cycle is irregular, 4) Non-24-Hour Sleep-Wake Type, where the cycle runs longer than 24 hours and does not reset with zeitgebers like morning daylight. 5) Shift Work Type is an inability to change sleep hours needed for shift work. 6) Due to medical conditions in which a sickness like flu when someone is bedridden, hospitalization (ICU), or use of drugs like stimulants can alter the circadian rhythm.

Jet Lag is a normal condition and people generally adjust to 2-hour changes per day. For example, if we travel across an 8-hour time zone, it would take 4 days to reset the circadian clock. Some have difficulty in adjusting to the change.

Treatment for circadian rhythm disturbances involve chronotherapy in which, the sleep hours are assigned to change it progressively by 3 hours per day. Light therapy with 10,000 lux natural light is useful in adjusting the body clock. Using body temperature which reaches its lowest point in the early morning, the light can be used to wake up and train the body to get used to the appropriate cycle. For example, early morning exposure to bright light can advance the cycle in late sleepers and evening light therapy can help early sleepers to stay up late and adjust to the new cycle. Light therapy may help jet lag, shift workers, and astronauts. Melatonin secretes as the night falls and as we close the eyes, and it stops secreting upon waking up and daylight. Melatonin is successfully used in circadian rhythm disturbances including jet lag.

Parasomnias

These include disorders with partial arousal such as sleepwalking, sleep-related eating, sexomnia or sexual acts during sleep, and sleep terrors are classified as NREM sleep arousal disorders.

Sleepwalking is common in 4-8-year olds and contrary to popular belief they are not dreaming or acting out the dreams, because this happens during NREM sleep. Sleepwalking ranges from just sitting up in bed to complex behaviors like driving, eating or having sexual acts. These may range from eating a snack or having something to drink, to eating elaborate meals. Sexomnia involves masturbation, fondling, or pelvic thrusting and rarely intercourse or even sexual assault. The sleepwalkers are partially awake and not fully aware of what they are doing. They may avoid obstacles but exhibit poor judgment (e.g.) urinating in the closet or walking out the window. There is no proven treatment for the parasomnias. The children usually grow out of sleep walking. Waking them up during a sleepwalk may terrify them or confuse them, but they need to be calmly redirected to the bed. A wet blanket near bed that wakes them up when they step on it, bells or even electric shocks are used to make the behavior go away, but nothing is proven to help reliably. Sedatives and sleep hygiene are tried with variable success rates.

Parasomnias Associated with REM Sleep

1. REM sleep behavior disorder: the individual is not able to have the sleep paralysis or loss of muscle tone that occurs during REM. They end up acting out their dreams which may be dangerous. The individual is not aware of the surroundings as they act out the context of the dream.

2. Recurrent isolated sleep paralysis may be associated with narcolepsy. A conscious mind and a "paralyzed body" even for a minute or two can be terrifying. It can happen in normal individuals under stress or poor sleep.

3. Nightmares: these are terrifying dreams that can occur frequently causing poor sleep. They are common in PTSD, personality disorders and schizophrenia. Sedatives, and antidepressants can help. Prazosin (1 or 2 mg), a central alpha-adrenergic antagonist is a popular treatment for PTSD related nightmares.

Restless Leg Syndrome (RLS)

RLS is a strong urge to keep the legs moving or shaking, especially when resting or trying to fall asleep. Patients have a strong urge to move their legs and give in by walking out of the bed for relief while they try to fall asleep. They may do this to a point that their sleep gets disturbed significantly. Causes include, iron deficiency anemia, diabetes, rheumatoid arthritis, Parkinson's disease, fibromyalgia, thyroid disease and COPD. It gets better with the treatment of the underlying cause. Dopamine agonists, pramipexole (Mirapex) and ropinirole (Mirapex), levodopa, benzodiazepines and gabapentin show benefit.

Bruxism

Teeth grinding in sleep is very common and is estimated to be prevalent from 8% to 31% in the general population, and if jaw clenching and milder or occasional teeth grinding are included, about 80% are estimated to be affected. This can lead to excessive dental wear, hypersensitive teeth and other dental problems. Bruxism can also happen during the daytime when individuals are awake. It is treated with reassurance, dental guards or occlusal splints to reduce the wear on the teeth. CBT and treatment of any associated sleep problems or stress might help.

Chapter 16

Sexual Disorders

Human Sexuality

Love and sex are unquestionably the most universal topics of interest for everyone. For any organism, procreation is the second most important function after survival. Living things evolved because they survived and procreated[1]. Understandably, hunger and the need for procreation are very basic functions and are represented in the older or primitive parts of the brain. In addition, evolution has reinforced behaviors related to sex and food associating with pleasure. Romantic love or passionate love, sexual act (with or without love) and compassionate non-romantic love share brain networks and involve a variety of neurochemicals including but is not limited to dopamine, serotonin, oxytocin and cortisol.

While sex may be experienced without love, they are psychologically and biologically associated functions. A primal source of pleasure and satisfaction, love and sex can also bring much pain, suffering and stress. In fact, the brain and body perceive and react to falling in love like it would react in a stressful situation by secreting cortisol and activating the body more or less like the fight or flight mode. Such activation, along with the cortisol, leads to the increased heart rate, sweaty palms and anxiety. Falling in love activates the dopamine mediated reward circuit in the brain[2]. It is the same area that gets activated with

---

[1] Almost everything we do can be traced back to these functions. Interestingly, the female orgasm has been an enigma for evolutionary biologists because it may not be necessary for procreation. It is believed to be a remnant of evolution. Without female orgasm or pleasure sexual act could be less interesting for men also end up as an abuse.

[2] The mesolimbic dopaminergic circuit from Ventral Tegmental Area (VTA) to the Nucleus Accumbens (NAc), as part of the Median Forebrain Bundle (MFB) is referred as the Hedonic Highway, and is considered as the most important reward circuit in the brain. Dopamine secretion in the VTA tags an experience as pleasurable (or aversive)

alcohol, cocaine, food and even video games. The high dopamine is probably responsible for the good feeling, acute focus, and heightened sense of awareness. Drugs that increase dopamine in the reward circuit, such as stimulants increase sexual desire and amorous pleasure. The anxiety and neurotic obsession about the other person are suspected to be associated with low serotonin. Lower serotonin is also associated with orgasm.

Oxytocin, sometimes called the "love hormone," is a peptide synthesized in hypothalamus and secreted in the posterior pituitary. Oxytocin enables the ejection of milk in lactating mothers, and the uterine contraction during childbirth. It is believed that oxytocin is behind the mother's "rush" of love towards the baby and secretes when fathers hold or play with the baby. Believed to secrete with touch, hugging or cuddling, oxytocin plays an important role in social behavior, trust and bonding. It's role in sex and orgasm is unclear, but it is suspected that it is part of the overall good feeling that comes with love and sex (along with dopamine and other monoamines). Oxytocin and vasopressin are believed to help us establish long term bonding and compassion.

Love is sometimes differentiated as passionate love and compassionate love. Passionate love is the experience of falling in love or being "in love" with someone fueled by sexual desire or desire for intimacy, and compassionate love is the "regular" kind of love that is predominantly a care for the other person. A romantic relationship that may start with passionate love may transform into compassionate love over a period of time, which married couples may perceive as a failure or loss of romantic interest. However, recent research supports the idea that the passionate love can be rekindled even decades after marriage. After all, the circuits and hormones are there - they just need to be retooled and reconditioned.

Sex (meaning sexual intercourse in this context), as raw and primitive as it seems is a masterfully orchestrated amalgamation of psychological, physiological, physical and neurological aspects of the body and self. The feeling of love and care buildup desire and prime us for sex. Sexual activity is described in four phases: excitation, plateau, orgasm and resolution. The central and autonomic nervous systems are involved in the sexual activity. The same areas explained above as the

---

mediated through NAc. Hippocampus helps form memories and amygdala helps tag those memories with emotion (pleasure in this context). The hypothalamus helps with physiological control of the body and the prefrontal cortex enables the person to seek or avoid pleasure or pain. Understandably, this reward circuit is a very primitive area in terms of evolution. Even some flies and worms that evolved a billion years ago have dopamine mediated reward circuits.

pleasure circuit is involved in sex[3]. Dopamine, glutamic acid, nitric oxide (vasodilation and erection), oxytocin and ACTH facilitate the sexual activity and serotonin, gamma-aminobutyric acid (GABA) and opioid reduce it. Alcohol stimulates the pleasure circuit, suppresses cortical inhibition (and impairs judgment or decision-making process in the choice of a mate), and increases the desire for sex, but its GABA like inhibition also impairs the performance.

Excitation involves erection and seminal secretion in men and vaginal lubrication and clitoral erection in women. Plateau is the time between excitement and orgasm while the sexual act continues. Plateau primes the genitalia for orgasm. For men, the erection stabilizes, and testicles move up in the scrotum. In women, the clitoris becomes very sensitive and even painful for touch and the vagina engorges with blood. Male orgasm consists of ejaculation and rapid contractions of penile muscles, prostate and anal sphincter that lasts for about 3 to 10 seconds. Female orgasm involves contraction of the uterus, vagina, pelvic muscles and anal sphincter lasting for 20 seconds or more. The resolution phase in men lasts for about 20 minutes to several hours during which period they cannot experience another orgasm, but women do not have this resolution phase, and so, are able to experience prolonged orgasm or multiple orgasms. Women report relaxation following orgasm, which corresponds to PET imaging finding of reduced blood flow to orbitofrontal cortex, amygdala and hippocampus. However, while majority of men report orgasm during sex, only a fraction of women reports orgasm, and some even report never experiencing orgasms.

Dopamine and oxytocin are involved in orgasm. In addition to exciting the pleasure circuit, orgasm inhibits the lateral orbitofrontal cortex, which controls emotions, self-evaluation, and reason. The anterior cingulate cortex orchestrates hormonal control of sex and sexual arousal. Sex related behavior including controlling the impulse, and processing sexual stimuli, are controlled by the cortex. The limbic system is involved in sexual arousal and the brainstem exerts control over peripheral sexual organs through pelvic efferent neurons using serotonin, which inhibits or delays orgasm. Dopamine inhibits prolactin secretion, which dampens the sexual response. However, low prolactin level is also associated with poor sexual functioning in men. Dopamine blocking antipsychotics increase prolactin and the SSRIs increase serotonin influencing sexual behavior.

Developmentally, sexual behavior starts early. Infants engage in genital play as part of the exploration of their bodies. As they grow, the

---

3 It has been found that sexually rejected male drosophila (fruit flies) resort to drinking alcohol heavily - should sound familiar to some male readers.

interest gets subdued for a while before coming back roaring during adolescence with the hormones. Sexual identity is decided by the sex chromosome with XY as male and XX as female. Chromosomal abnormalities such as Turner's syndrome (single X in sex chromosome or XO) lead to ambiguous external and internal genitalia, causing problems with gender identity.

Gender Identity is defined as the psychological aspect of behavior related to masculinity or femininity. Gender identity is "assigned" by the appearance of the external genitalia and essentially given to the individual by the family, society and culture. However, the individual needs to develop a gender identity for himself or herself, which may not always coincide with the anatomy. Sexual orientation is the inherent propensity of the individual's romantic and sexual attraction towards a certain gender.

Sexual behavior is driven by the biological forces, but environment and culture play a major role. Cultural, societal and religious expectation of sexual behavior influences its learning during developmental years, which varies tremendously between sexes - sometimes the cause of misogyny. It is believed that, considering the evolutionary principles, and the gender difference in the biology, men are driven to have more sex and, so, procreate more. Whereas, women are driven to protect the baby and its wellbeing. Thus, men have higher baseline desire, and are easily excitable by simple visual cues. Whereas, women are careful and cautious, with lower level of desire, needing reassurance, comfort, and safety (to care for the baby), and are aroused by emotional cues.

Thus, men are attracted by the appearance of voluptuous women with wide hips, and bigger mammary glands (which, technically, is supposed to reassure the man that his offspring will be well fed and increase the chance of survival). Women are attracted to gallant hero who happens to be passionately and hopelessly in love with her, so that he would stay with her, protect her and her offspring for years to come. As the humans evolved, and modern societies formed, these biological differences influenced the sexual behavior. The religious, legal, and societal norms are developed based on these principles. The taboos against premarital and extramarital sex, homosexuality, incest, and even masturbation, evolved from these sex differences.

DSM-5 lists 10 sexual disorders that are more or less self-explanatory. The clinical features and diagnosis are not complex. The major issue is that the patients typically do not easily talk to clinicians about their sexual problems due to the private nature of the behavior and the general cultural sentiments. Many cultures and religions venerate celibacy and discourage hedonic sexual behavior. Sexual health is significantly intertwined to mental health as many mental illnesses and their treatment affect intimacy and sex.

Treatment of sexual disorders is mostly nonspecific involving education, reassurance and support. There are a lot of myths and misconceptions about sex that influence the sexual behavior. Considering the complexity of the sexual behavior, an evaluation of the patient should include psychological, behavioral, biological, cultural aspects. Many factors from religion-based ideas, hygiene, personal attitudes, relationship issues and medications should be addressed.

Male Hypoactive Sexual Disorder

This is defined as a lack of sexual thoughts, fantasies and desire for sex, or in short, lack of desire (which might seem to be a relief for some men). It varies with age; 6% in young men and 40% in men over 65.

Female Sexual Interest/Arousal Disorder

Sexual interest and arousal are combined in women because stimulation and arousal with vaginal lubrication occur with desire in most women. Women are not as preoccupied as men about sex, although they also involve in sexual fantasies with a strong romantic overtone. A reduction in the interest and arousal is characterized in this disorder. Flibanserin (Addyi, 100 mg taken once a day at bedtime), a serotonin agonist and Bremelanotide (Vyleesi), a melanocortin receptor agonist (1.75mg injected subcutaneously) are approved by the FDA to help improve libido in women.

Erectile Disorder

Inability to have an erection, commonly known as impotence can be psychological or biological. It is usually more psychological in the young, and more organic or biological in the old. Many men are petrified by the thought of impotence, which can increase the anxiety and perpetuate the problem. A number of psychological factors that are interpersonal in nature between the man and his partner such as love, desire, anger and trust can influence the erection. Men could feel helpless and powerless when they face erectile disorder. With the recent advent of PDE5 inhibitors (Sildenafil (Viagra), tadalafil (Cialis)) and their marketing campaign has reassured and "invigorated" middle aged men. It is estimated that about half of the men above the age 50 have some erectile dysfunction. Although vascular reasons are cited, psychological factors can certainly play a role. Observing erection during REM sleep is evidence that the biological mechanism involved in erection is intact.

Female Orgasmic Disorder

5% to 10% of women never experienced orgasm and some are actually not distressed about it[4]. Female orgasmic disorder or anorgasmia may be primary (never had one) or acquired. A number of psychological issues ranging from feelings about men or a partner, body image, or sociocultural attitudes about sex can influence her capacity to enjoy sex. No pharmacotherapy has been well established. Some women report better sex with PDE5 inhibitors, but the clinical evidence is not strong, and it is not FDA approved.

Delayed Ejaculation

This is characterized by difficulty in reaching orgasm with coitus. Antidepressants such as SSRIs can cause this, but most of the times, it is reflective of interpersonal issues between the man and his partner. Sometimes, men may not be able to reach orgasm, even in the presence of ejaculation. Delay in ejaculation happening occasionally can be normal, but as it gets chronic it can be very annoying and frustrating. It is estimated that 3% to 5% of men have this condition, and it is believed that this may become more common due to the widely available pornography in the internet. It is hypothesized that excessive pornography desensitizes and alters ideas and attitudes about sex. It has also been reported that neuronal connections in the brain could be different for those who are exposed to excessive pornography. Treatment would include addressing the underlying cause and psychotherapy.

Premature Ejaculation

Reaching orgasm before it is intended is a common complaint among men. This may actually be a more common or frequent concern of men than impotence. However, men can lose track of the time and may have unrealistic expectations about their performance. The "performance" or the duration of copulation may also be influenced by edited pornography giving an appearance of excessively long performance. Orgasm or ejaculation within one minute of penetration is considered premature ejaculation. It is estimated to be prevalent at 1-3%. Use of SSRIs to delay ejaculation is becoming more popular, but anorgasmia can become an issue. Kegel's exercise is recommended to help prolong the performance. A good majority of men might benefit from a thorough and realistic evaluation and reassurance. A reduction in performance

---

4 In fact, the evolutionary significance of female orgasm has been a highly debated topic of intellectual curiosity. Female orgasm may not be necessary for the preservation of the species, but female biology may not be distinct enough to differentiate orgasm compared to childbearing and childbirth. Yet, without the pleasure, women could perceive sex as a chore or could feel abused.

anxiety by having realistic expectations helps many patients. A major culprit is alcohol, which may dampen the performance.

Interestingly, the goal of sex (besides the procreation) is to reach an orgasm, and, considering the fact that women have more orgasms with masturbation than penile stimulation, educating the couple about aspects of sex and foreplay without the insertion of penis in the vagina, may help reduce the anxiety related to performance. Squeeze technique involves stimulation of the penis to a point of early signs of ejaculation and at that point, if the coronal ridge of the glans penis is squeezed it would reduce the erection and prevent ejaculation. Stop-start technique also involves something similar in which the sexual stimulation of the penis is conducted until the point of early signs of ejaculation, stop the stimulation, wait until the erection comes down and the feeling of impending climax disappears and then continue the act. This is essentially training the penis to wait, and it needs patience and discipline. Some claim that men who masturbate regularly to achieve a quick ejaculation and orgasm may have inadvertently trained their penises for a quick ejaculation. There is a huge underground market in "performance enhancement" which in actuality may allay the fears and anxiety around the performance than improve the performance.

Genito-pelvic Pain/Penetration Disorder

These include dyspareunia and vaginismus. Dyspareunia is pain in the vagina during copulation caused by partial contraction of the vaginal wall (muscles involved are bulbocavernosus, transverse perineal, ischiocavernosus, and levator ani) which may have organic causes like infection or psychological. Vaginismus is a severe contraction of these muscles resulting in a difficulty to insert penis or finger. Ruling out organic causes would be the first step in treatment, especially in acquired dyspareunia or vaginismus. Psychological factors may include fear of sex, fear of pain (especially the first time), and interpersonal relationship issues. The woman's attitude towards sex and her partner must be evaluated for conflicts. Reassurance, relaxation and conflict resolution would help.

Substance/Medication induced Sexual Dysfunction

A number of drugs can influence sex by interfering with desire, arousal, performance and orgasm. Psychiatric drugs are major culprits. This is due to the influence on neurotransmitters in the central and peripheral nervous systems. Antipsychotics can interfere with sex by increasing prolactin secretion. Drugs that increase serotonin causes decreased drive and anorgasmia, drugs with anticholinergic activity interfere with erection and ejaculation. Stimulants increase the sex drive, at least initially. Alcohol and other "downers" like benzodiazepines and opioids may increase the desire by disinhibition or reduce the anxiety around sex, thus improving the performance, but in general, they dampen the enthusiasm and interfere with performance.

Other specified Sexual Dysfunction

Postcoital Dysphoria: As opposed to feeling relaxed, and content, some may feel anxiety, fear or sadness after sex. This is common among men and in the context of guilt or fear associated with the sexual act.

Postcoital headache: common among women. Sometimes migraines and cluster headaches can be precipitated by coitus.

Persistent sexual arousal disorder: Rare condition seen in some women with schizophrenia. Affected women have continuous arousal and masturbate incessantly for relief. They do not report excessive desire or interest in having sex. It is a relief of a tension as opposed to a pleasure

Unspecified Sexual Dysfunction includes any sexual dysfunction not described above.

Treatment of Sexual Dysfunction

Dual-sex Therapy

Pioneered by Masters and Johnson in Indiana, this involves a four-way round table discussion of the sexual practices by the couple with a team of male and female therapists. But, in practice, most often only a single therapist is involved. The therapist would evaluate in detail about the sexual practices, knowledge, preferences, relationship issues, attitudes towards sex, conflicts and other problems. Any organic cause of the problem is also evaluated and addressed. Most of the times, the patient's problems stem from inadequate knowledge, misinformation, misconception, and unrealistic expectation or anxiety over performance. Specific recommendations and exercises are offered to improve the sexual functioning with an emphasis on communication, romance, foreplay and education of non-penetration aspects of sex.

The treatment involves education, reassurance and anxiety reduction. Marital discord, communication problems and other interpersonal issues are usually the most important causes of poor satisfaction in sex. Relaxation techniques and CBT can reduce anxiety. CBT principles of desensitization and anxiety reduction can be applied in sex therapy. The patients make a list of anxiety provoking events related to sex and are encouraged to perform and practice those acts from least anxiety provoking events (touching or kissing) to most anxiety provoking behavior (penetration). Mindfulness therapy directing the couple to enjoy the moment instead of watching, analyzing and judging their performance, referred to as "spectating," will help them have a more pleasurable experience. Group therapies where couples find that some issues are common and not to be feared over are also very effective.

Medications Used in Sex Therapy

PDE5 inhibitors: introduction of sildenafil (Viagra, and others since then tadalafil (Cialis) and vardenafil (Levitra)) and associated marketing campaigns revolutionized sex in the elderly. These drugs enhance the action of nitric oxide (NO) which is essential for erection. NO activates the enzyme guanylate cyclase, which results in an increase in cyclic guanosine monophosphate (cGMP). PDE5 inhibitors inhibit degradation of cGMP, leading to better erection from sexual stimulation. PDE5 inhibitors are not reported to be beneficial in women but they increase the lubrication and improves blood flow to the clitoris. Since the advent of PDE5 inhibitors, other drugs described here have lost popularity. The discovery of the role of nitric oxide in the blood vessels (not exactly about erection) led to a Nobel Prize[5].

Phentolamine: an alpha-adrenergic antagonist that causes vasodilatation and erection. Available as pills or injection.

Apomorphine: a dopamine agonist that is believed to increase desire in men, but the proof is not convincing.

Alprostadil (prostaglandin E1): This is a naturally occurring prostaglandin E1. It is injected directly on the shaft of the penis and causes immediate erection that lasts for about two hours. A topical cream and urethral suppository are also available.

Papaverine is an opioid alkaloid present in poppy plant. It is a smooth muscle relaxer and it can cause erection when injected in the penis.

Bromocriptine: is an ergot derivative and a dopamine agonist. It can counter the increased prolactin level caused by antipsychotics.

Trazodone is known to improve nocturnal erection, but its clinical utility is unclear.

Ginseng: Some believe that it can improve sexual health, but the evidence is not convincing.

Yohimbine: This is a naturally occurring alkaloid that blocks alpha 2 adrenergic receptors and causes vasodilation. It was considered as a possible cure for ED, but the introduction of PDE5 inhibitors has made this less popular.

---

5 1998 Nobel Prize for physiology and medicine was awarded to Robert F. Furchgott, Louis J. Ignarro and Ferid Murad for their work in the discovery of the role of NO as a vasodilator.

Drugs with stimulant properties: cocaine, amphetamines, cannabis, and hallucinogens are reported to improve all aspects of sex including the subjective experience. The reaction to drugs by individuals varies and many people can experience an increase in anxiety, fear and paranoia. Chronic and regular use can lead to poor sexual health.

Hormones

Androgen: Testosterone increases sex drive in women and men - especially in the presence of low testosterone levels. Women can develop virilizing side effects such as facial hair growth, and men can develop hypertension or prostate problems. It is not an entirely safe option.

Estrogen: Estrogen administration as part of birth control can reduce libido. Locally applied estrogen as a vaginal cream, ring or a tablet can improve arousal and lubrication.

Clomiphene and tamoxifen act as antiestrogens and induce secretion of gonadotropin releasing hormone and increase testosterone level which increases libido in women.

Vacuum pump: Elderly men and patients after prostate surgery used to be prescribed this simple vacuum pump to fill blood into penis to cause an erection. This is not popular since the advent of PDE5 inhibitors.

Male prosthesis: A semi rigid rod or an inflatable can be implanted that gives a permanent or temporary augmentation of erection.

Sex Addiction

This is not a diagnosis in DSM-5 but based on the concept of addiction to drugs or gambling, people who spend excessive amounts of time for sex and sex related activities, whose life revolves around the next sexual act, and those who want to and try to cut down their sexual behavior because it bothers them can be described as addicted to sex. These individuals are generally unhappy with their need and are perturbed about the preoccupation and the time and effort spent on sex. Sex addiction can be associated with paraphilias or towards normal sexual behavior. Treatment is similar to the support groups based on the 12-step program: sex addicts anonymous.

Gender Dysphoria

Gender identity is the person's sense of maleness or femaleness which usually corresponds to the biological or assigned sex. Previously called as gender identity disorder, gender dysphoria implies a discomfort with the assigned or biological sex. Transgender include, transsexuals who want the body of the opposite sex, cross dressers are those who dress in the cloths of the opposite sex but retain their assigned gender, genderqueer are those who consider themselves in between, both or neither gender. The DSM-5 has modified its approach in the diagnosis with an emphasis on dysphoria or distress as opposed to the idea of transgender itself. Similarly, it also makes it clear that only the children who clearly express their desire to be the opposite sex, and only those who are distressed about their assigned sex and expected gender related behavior of the assigned sex are considered transgender. Children who behave like they are opposite sex for a variety of reasons (wanting to dress like the opposite sex and a girl wanting to behave like her brother - tomboy) are not considered a problem. Even those children who are accepted and supported to live as the chosen gender and feel comfortable in the non-assigned gender are not diagnosed with gender dysphoria. In addition, DSM-5 moves away from the binary male - female differentiation of gender and emphasizes on the distress. The cross-gender behavior itself, without any distress, is not diagnosed as a disorder.

Gender dysphoria is a rare condition with a prevalence of 1 in 11,000 to 30,000 men or 1 in 30,000 to 100,000 women. All fetuses start as female and sexual differentiation occurs or differentiation as a male happens, only by the influence of fetal androgen. The short arm of Y chromosome has a gene referred to as SRY (Sex-determining Region of Y) which is responsible for the testicle determining factor (TDF) which in turn, differentiates the gonadal tissue of the fetus into testes. This happens at around 6-8 weeks of gestation. Without TDF or Y chromosome, the fetus would develop into a female phenotype. The exposure or lack of it, of the fetus to sex hormones is suspected to influence the gender dysphoria but the evidence is not convincing. However, any abnormalities in the exposure, or lack of it, can lead to ambiguous genitalia which can lead to issues with gender identity.

Psychosocial aspects of gender roles, identity and behavior are hotly debated topics, especially in rearing children. It is possible that children's gender specific behavior is somewhat biologically based, and to some extent, learned. A mild cross gender behavior is common among growing children. Gender specific behavior starts before age 3, and some children may report discomfort with the assigned gender or report a desire to be the opposite gender even at that age. While some individuals "know" early on and grow up to become transgender individuals, not all children with gender dysphoria grow up to transgender individuals. Conversely, some adult transgender people do not report or recall gender dysphoria growing up. It is also true that not all transgender people feel "trapped in the body of opposite sex." The gender identity seems to be a continuum from female to male, and people fall in any end of the spectrum with most men feeling manly and most of the women feeling feminine - predominantly.

Treatment of gender dysphoria varies from reassurance to surgical and hormonal therapies to achieve primary and secondary sexual characteristics of the opposite sex, if desired. Such an intervention may start at an early age, sometimes even in kindergarten. As the child reaches puberty, this may be time to intervene hormonally or surgically to modify the sex, if the child desires. Such a drastic change involves complete evaluation by a team of professionals before making the decision. Mental health is assessed as a requirement and transgender individuals are more susceptible for anxiety, depression, substance abuse, sexual abuse and self-injurious behavior. Transgender men with female anatomy can take a series of testosterone injections to gain masculine characteristics. Transgender women with male anatomy can take estrogen, testosterone blockers, progesterone or usually a combination of these. Very few individuals resort to sex reassignment surgery, which may vary from relatively simple procedures (breast implant) to complex and expensive reconstructions.

Paraphilias

Paraphilias are sexual perversions that are deviant from the normal sexual behavior. There are some caveats in the diagnosis of paraphilias, meaning just a fantasy of a deviant act in itself does not constitute an illness. The individual needs to feel that the deviant acts are necessary for sexual arousal and orgasm. These deviant impulses need to be expressed behaviorally meaning they act out their fantasies and their sexual behavior is restricted to the perversion. When they do not act on those impulses, they should cause marked distress and interference in day to day life.

Paraphilias can involve aggression, victimization, and one-sided acts forced on others like rape or sexual abuse of children. The deviant fantasy or rumination is the pathognomonic feature of paraphilia. Acting upon them to derive pleasure, satisfaction or relief would reinforce and perpetuate the deviant behavior. The one-sided nature of paraphilias defeat the purpose of love and sex as enablers of bonding. Victims of paraphilia are severely traumatized, and a single individual with deviant behavior, such as pedophilia can traumatize hundreds of victims.

Paraphilias are more common in men, start before age 18, peak around age 25 and it is uncommon after age 50. Individuals with one paraphilia often have other related illnesses. Classic psychoanalytic thinking supposes that the normal sexual development is interfered with, resulting in paraphilia. Learning theory supports the idea of developing paraphilias from modeling and mimicking from the media or personal experiences. Pedophilia, or sexual interest towards children, is the most common paraphilia. It has been noted that many individuals with pedophilia used to be victims of sexual abuse as children, supporting both psychoanalytic developmental and learning theories. Some studies have identified a few biological abnormalities including hormonal and chromosomal abnormalities. It appears that these are more biologically based abnormalities.

Specific paraphilias

Exhibitionism: Men exposing their genitals to unsuspecting women to get aroused or to reach an orgasm during or right after the exposure with or without masturbation.

Fetishism: Exclusively found in men who get aroused with objects such as shoes, panties and stockings. A similar focus on body parts such as feet is known as partialism.

Frotteurism: Again, exclusively male behavior of man rubbing his penis in the buttocks of a fully clothed, unsuspecting, woman. This happens in crowded public places like subways and buses.

Voyeurism: Preoccupation and fantasies about watching and observing unsuspecting women grooming, bathing, having sex or just being on their own in their privacy.

Sexual masochism: recurrent preoccupation, fantasies and urges involving being humiliated, tied up, beaten or otherwise made to suffer for the purpose of sexual arousal, orgasm or enhancement of sexual experience. Asphyxiophilia is a variant of masochism where the individual chokes himself, with or without help, to reach a level of asphyxia to obtain or enhance sexual arousal or orgasm.

Sexual sadism: Sexual arousal from the physical or psychological suffering of another person. Rape is not necessarily sadism because it involves a sense of power, but rape can be an aspect of sadism. People who rape and kill women (lust murders) are frequently mentally ill. Mental illness along with hormonal abnormalities, familial predisposition, pathological relationships, and history of sex abuse seem to contribute to this.

Transvestism: Wearing clothes of the opposite gender for sexual arousal, masturbation and orgasm. More common in men but can occur in women. May overlap with gender dysphoria. Some men may eventually prefer to wear and live in women's clothes.

Necrophilia is a desire to gratify sexual urges from a cadaver. *Zoophilia* is a desire to have sex with animals. *Coprophilia* is a desire to defecate on a partner or be defecated on and urophilia is a desire to urinate on a partner or be urinated upon. *Klismaphilia* is use of enema for erotic purposes.

A popular textbook of psychiatry lists masturbation in this section of paraphilia and reports it is normal. Oh well, masturbation *is* normal. What a relief!

Chapter 17

Psychopharmacology

Psychopharmacology is very simple. There are only a few classes of medications to study: antidepressants, antipsychotics, mood stabilizers, anxiolytics and stimulants. Among these, all stimulants are essentially derivatives of amphetamines, and behave the same way. Sleep medications and anxiolytics are similar, and considering the addiction potential, it is important to remember to use these drugs occasionally and for only a short period of time. This leaves just three groups of medications to study: antipsychotics, antidepressants, and mood stabilizers. If someone can master the use of these, they can manage almost any situation in psychiatry with medications, and put us, the psychiatrists, out of business.

Yet, psychopharmacology is not often that straightforward and at times confusing. Antidepressants, as the name implies, are helpful in depression, but they are also the main treatment of choice for anxiety disorders and OCD. In addition to treating psychosis, antipsychotics are the main treatment of choice for acute mania. Antipsychotics and mood stabilizers work for augmentation of bipolar depression. Comorbidities often lead to polypharmacy and confusion in treatment. Some bipolar patients, even when they are stable, may need a mood stabilizer, an antidepressant, and an antimanic, which is an antipsychotic - all at the same time.

One might see all three or four (or even five) classes of medications on the same patient. While this may not be entirely wrong, polypharmacy in general may reflect a difficult patient (difficult in terms of symptoms or cooperation), poor diagnosis, or poor management. A combination of stimulants and downers, or stimulants and antipsychotics, do not make any sense unless it is justified by the unique situation and explained clearly. Any sedative (including antihistamines) can impair the alertness and attention. It is sometimes hard to understand if someone takes a downer at night (with 24-hour action) and a stimulant during the day, basically engineering their cognition. An amphetamine-like-stimulant can cause or worsen psychosis and so, it rarely, if ever, makes sense for someone with psychosis to be on stimulants.

The most important aspect of psychopharmacology is diagnosis. A clear diagnosis and identification of a specific target symptom would help with precise treatment and appropriate choice of medication. An unclear diagnosis or target symptoms often leads to polypharmacy. The treatment of specific conditions is discussed in relevant chapters. Here, I will discuss some general principles of psychopharmacology, and list commonly used medications.

Although still far behind the rest of the medical field, treatment in mental health has made significant advances in the past 50 or 60 years. Nonetheless, there is still a long way to go, and cure for many conditions is still elusive. However, some chronic diseases like depression or generalized anxiety disorder can be controlled fairly adequately, and patients may be expected to live a relatively symptom free life.

Within classes of medications, there may not be major differences among the agents in terms of efficacy. Unlike antibiotics, superiority in efficacy of one medication over others within a specific class has not been well established, in general. However, the medications differ significantly in terms of side effects and so, the first choice is almost always made based on the potential side effects. Some side effects like sedation may be desirable in some situations. In addition, the choice may often be influenced by the bias of the patient or the clinician. Patients vary widely in the way they respond or tolerate a specific medication. So, the history of medication use is very important to keep in mind when you start someone on a new medication. The most important aspect to consider in treating any patient is cost benefit ratio and the ideal medication should treat the condition with no side effects.

Antipsychotics

Antipsychotics are used to treat psychosis of any kind, although they are typically studied and approved for schizophrenia. Chlorpromazine made history by being the first medication to treat psychosis and schizophrenia. It was synthesized in 1952 in France and was initially used for pre-anesthesia. Henri Laborit, a military surgeon, noticed its calming effect and persuaded his colleagues[1] to test it on a psychotic

---

1 The first patient to receive chlorpromazine for psychosis was a 24-year-old man named Jacques Lh. He was severely manic, psychotic and agitated. He was given 50 mg of chlorpromazine intravenously at 10 AM on January 19th of 1952. He apparently calmed down immediately but needed more injections. He developed problems in his veins due to the

patient. They discovered that the patient improved in his psychosis after pushing the dose to a total of 855 mg of chlorpromazine in 20 days, establishing the first ever treatment for psychosis. Later, the medication was studied in detail by Pierre Deniker and John Delay and was proven to be a viable antipsychotic medication.

Around this time, dopamine was discovered as a neurotransmitter and the idea of brain receptors and their role became popular and widely accepted. A lack of dopamine in the brain was attributed to Parkinson's disease and chlorpromazine was noted to cause stiffness and shakes similar to Parkinson's disease. Hence, dopamine blockade was believed to be the mechanism of action behind the chlorpromazine. As the understanding of this got better, and by putting two and two together, Jac Van Rossum proposed the Dopamine Hypothesis of Schizophrenia, implying an increase in dopamine is behind psychosis. Following this, a number of drugs that block dopamine, such as haloperidol were introduced. Dopamine blockage, while helped improve psychosis caused side effects called extrapyramidal symptoms or EPS. These dopamine blocking drugs are sometimes referred to as first generation antipsychotics.

Clozapine, now considered a "second generation" antipsychotic was discovered in 1960 and was shown to be effective for schizophrenia, nonetheless suspicion lingered around its efficacy as an antipsychotic because it did not cause EPS. It was first introduced in Austria and later in Germany in 1970. While it was immediately liked by psychiatrists as well as patients, the sale of the drug came to an absolute halt after a report of 16 patients developing an unusual side effect called agranulocytosis which was fatal in 8 of them. Agranulocytosis is a deficiency or reduction of granulocytes (white blood cells) which leads to susceptibility for infections and death. The reason behind the agranulocytosis is not fully understood; it is not an allergic reaction and can occur even after years of use. Because of such a risk, the US FDA made an unusual mandate that clozapine should be proven superior to other existing medications and insisted on a safety mechanism to identify and treat agranulocytosis. The drug was reintroduced in the USA with specific guidelines to monitor blood regularly, and patients were tracked in a national registry. Clozapine became very popular in the 90s because of the hope it presented for medication resistant patients. The popularity and use of clozapine have come down recently as several newer antipsychotics have been introduced in the market but, even now, a lot of

---

irritation from the drug. He was given barbiturates and electroshock treatment along with a series of injections of chlorpromazine. After a total of 855 mg of chlorpromazine in 20 days the patient improved and resumed normal life.

patients respond to clozapine when they fail to respond to other medications.

In recent years, a number of antipsychotic medications were introduced that are not direct dopamine blockers. Some of the newer antipsychotics have a different set of prominent side effects including weight gain and metabolic syndrome. The second-generation antipsychotics (SGA) are called atypical antipsychotics because they do not (often) cause EPS.

Most antipsychotics block postsynaptic dopamine D2 receptors. The SGAs bind to serotonin 5HT2 receptors more than dopamine D2 receptors, and this difference is suspected in the lesser EPS with SGAs. Some also believe that the SGAs bind and unbind with the receptor a lot more loosely than first generation antipsychotics or may attach to preferred receptors (more cognitive action than motor action) resulting in less EPS. Aripiprazole and brexpiprazole are dopamine D2 receptor partial agonists, and cariprazine is a dopamine D3/D2 receptor partial agonist. Partial agonists bind more preferably to the receptors than dopamine but are less effective than dopamine and so the net result is similar to a blockade. It is believed that all antipsychotics need to block dopamine D2 receptors, binding at about 65%, for antipsychotic efficacy.

Commonly Used Antipsychotics

Among the older antipsychotics only haloperidol is still widely used. Fluphenazine and chlorpromazine are prescribed less often. Other antipsychotics including, loxapine, molindone, pimozide, thioridazine, are rarely used and I do not suspect a reader of this book to ever use it. Haloperidol and fluphenazine are available as long acting injections. First generation antipsychotics in general have strong dopamine D2 blockade and common side effects include EPS, sedation, hyperprolactinemia, weight gain, and akathisia.

First Generation Antipsychotics		
Drug	Usual daily dose (daily max)	Half-life
Chlorpromazine (Thorazine, Largactil)	75 to 300 mg oral (1000mg); 25 to 50mg every 6 to 8 hrs as injection.	20 to 40 hours.
Haloperidol (Dozic, Haldol, Serenace)	1 to 4.5mg three times by mouth (20mg) – can be given once a day at bed time 2 to 5 mg by injection (12mg).	20 hours

First Generation Antipsychotics		
Fluphenazine (Prolixin)	2 to 10 mg (40mg)	35 hours
Long acting injections		
Haloperidol	25-200 mg IM once in 4 weeks	
Fluphenazine	25-100 mg IM once in two weeks.	

Second Generation Antipsychotics		
Drug	Usual daily dose (daily max)	Half-life in hours
Clozapine	100-700 mg in divided doses (800)	6-26
Risperidone	1-6 mg a day (12)	24
Paliperidone	3-12 mg a day (12)	23
Olanzapine	5-15 mg a day (20)	32+
Quetiapine	300-800 in divided doses (800)	7-12
Ziprasidone	40-160 taken twice a day (160)	7
Asenapine	5-20 Sublingual (20)	24
Lurasidone	37 to 148 mg (148)	20-40
Iloperidone	1-12 mg a day (12)	18-23
Aripiprazole	5-20 (30)	75-146
Brexpiprazole	0.25 -4mg (4)	91
Cariprazine	1.5-6 (6)	48-120

Long acting injections of SGA		
Risperidone	25 mg to 50 mg once in two weeks.	Three week overlap with oral medication is recommended
Paliperidone (monthly)	Available in 39, 78, 117, 156 and 234 mg	2-week overlap recommended

Long acting injections of SGA		
Paliperidone (3month preparation)	Available in 273, 410, 546, and 819 mg	
Aripiprazole monohydrate	300 or 400 mg per month	
Aripiprazole luroxil	441, 662, 882 mg per month (882 can be given q 6 weeks)	
Olanzapine	210, 300, 405 mg once a month	Not popular due to post injection observation requirement for post injection delirium, sedation syndrome.

Antipsychotic induced side effects

Extra Pyramidal Symptoms (EPS)

Extrapyramidal symptoms, commonly referred to as EPS occur frequently with the first-generation antipsychotics. EPS was a distinct and early side effect of antipsychotics and, as mentioned above, the discovery for new antipsychotics was focused on the molecule's ability to cause EPS, a side effect!

Muscle movements are controlled by several different areas of the brain. To understand in simple terms, the motor cortex sends the stimulus via the pyramidal tract that makes the muscle contract. The subcortical system helps in the smooth initiation and control of the muscle contractions to produce the intended movements of a ballet dancer or a tennis player. As the motor fibers descend from the brain, they look like a pyramid and so are called pyramidal fibers or pyramidal columns. The subcortical control of the dexterity does not involve these pyramidal fibers and so is known as "ExtraPyramidal." Acute Dystonias, Akathisia and Tardive Dyskinesia are the common EPS side effects to keep in mind.

Acute Dystonia

This is an immediate reaction of the antipsychotics, frequently seen after an injection of haloperidol or dopamine blocking antiemetics like metoclopramide (Reglan). The patient develops intense muscle spasms in any part of the body, but frequently in the jaw, neck and extremities. This is one of the most dramatic and grotesque side effects one can see in medicine. Fortunately, an administration of anticholinergic injection would immediately reduce or relieve the spasm[2].

Akathisia

Akathisia is a feeling of restlessness or an inability to sit still. The patients frequently report this as an anxiety but when asked "Do you feel like you cannot sit down and feel like you need to get up and go?" they usually recognize this as a restlessness. Something in the initiation of the movements goes wrong. It is sort of the opposite of Parkinson's disease where the initiation of the movement is difficult or delayed when a patient wants to get up and go. The patients describe this as an inner restlessness. When this occurs to agitated patients, it may become a bigger clinical problem. The best treatment for akathisia is to reduce the dose of the medication or change the medication. Propranolol helps in calming down. Benzodiazepines may be used in the acute setting. Anticholinergics are not very effective but are used commonly.

Parkinsonism

As the name implies, this presents more or less like Parkinson's disease. The patients exhibit the typical tremor, rigidity, bradykinesia and postural instability. The tremor is a rhythmic and repetitive movement of the extremities, sometimes referred to as "pill rolling movement" of the hands. The rigidity or stiffness leads to the stooped posture and a specific condition called cogwheel rigidity. Examining their joint movements, one can notice the staggered stiffness, typically at the elbow or wrist, which feels like moving the joint through a gear or a cogwheel. They also show mask like face, stooped posture and difficulty in initiat-

[2] The author had the unfortunate experience of witnessing such a morbid acute dystonia as a young and naive medical student. That too on his very first clinic day! As he happened to pass the crowded hallway of the hospital, he witnessed this poor young woman, being half carried by her family. She couldn't walk and could not even hold her clothes to save her modesty. Her body was contorted in a crooked manner with the jaw, neck and hands stretched and pulling in awkward directions. She had an eerie and painful expression, with the eyes rolled up and a steady drool dripping down her mouth. She was held at the arm by two people who literally dragged her as she struggled to walk. As yours truly concluded that moment that he made the gravest mistake by entering into medical school and as he decided to quit and walk away, his curiosity made him follow her to the injection clinic where she was promptly given an intramuscular injection. Voila! There she was! Back to normal but for the utter embarrassment. All the contortions and contractions disappeared like magic except the magician was wearing a white coat instead of a high hat. She walked away briskly avoiding the kind and fearful stares of the onlookers including the author. By this time, the author was totally conflicted with the fear of facing such cases and with the fantasy of becoming the nonchalant hero who gave the injection.

ing movements. This is an immediate side effect that would get better or disappear upon a reduction or stoppage of the medication. Anticholinergic medications such as trihexyphenidyl (Artane) or benztropine (Cogentin) 1 mg or 2 mg once or twice a day may relieve these symptoms.

Tardive dyskinesia (TD)

This is one of the most disabling side effects of antipsychotic use. Frequently referred to as TD, it happens after months or years of use of antipsychotics, and so is called "tardive." Unfortunately, this seems to result from a rather (seemingly) permanent damage of the brain and does not improve or change upon the discontinuation of the antipsychotics. TD is characterized by non-rhythmic, gyrating, chorea like movements in the tongue, jaw, limbs, or trunk. The movements appear almost purposeful, as if someone is chewing gum or smacking the lips. Sometimes TD gets worse after stopping the antipsychotics. In fact, some patients develop TD after aripiprazole is stopped known as withdrawal emergent TD. Women and patients who do not have schizophrenia seem to have a higher risk of developing TD. It is also been found to be associated with the use of metoclopramide. There are two new medications, valbenazine (40 or 80mg a day) and deutetrabenazine (6mg a day up to 48mg a day maximum), both VAMT2 inhibitors and derivatives of an old medication tetrabenazine introduced recently for the treatment of TD.

Metabolic Syndrome

Metabolic syndrome denotes a combination of significant weight gain or obesity, high triglycerides, high cholesterol along with an increase in insulin level. With obesity, these patients would be at a higher risk for diabetes, hypertension and coronary artery diseases. This is a common problem with some second-generation antipsychotics such as clozapine, olanzapine and quetiapine but can also happen with first generation antipsychotics also. Some drugs like aripiprazole, ziprasidone and asenapine seem to be weight neutral or do not cause significant weight gain.

QT Prolongation

Several psychiatric medications including chlorpromazine, haloperidol, risperidone, thioridazine, ziprasidone, and tricyclic antidepressants increase the QT interval in the ECG. An increase in the QT interval increases the risk of a cardiac arrhythmia called torsade de pointes which is life threatening. Although many medications, psychiatric and non-psychiatric can cause QT prolongation, ziprasidone, it seems, has been singled out for this side effect. Interestingly, there is no clear and convincing proof of torsades or death from ziprasidone. Yet, there is a prevailing fear with ziprasidone which might have unfairly curbed its use and sales[3]. However, this is a serious side effect that needs to be kept in mind, especially if the patient has a known history of prolonged QT interval.

Neuroleptic Malignant Syndrome

A serious side effect of antipsychotic medications that may be life threatening. It is characterized by high fever, muscle rigidity and confusion. Pulse and blood pressure may increase uncontrollably. Rhabdomyolysis, renal failure, hyperkalemia or seizures can happen. Treatment includes stopping the offending medications and cooling the patient. Dantrolene (for muscle relaxation), bromocriptine (reduce the effect of dopamine blockade) or diazepam may be needed.

Antidepressants

For a long time, even while mental illnesses were starting to be understood as brain disorders, depression and anxiety were perceived, at least by some, as the problems of the psyche or result of some internal psychological conflict, making the idea of treatment with medications untenable. Then, there were other misleading distinctions such as reactive depression and endogenous depression (sometimes referred to as minor and major depression). Reactive implies feeling sad because something bad happened, and endogenous implies that it is more biological, for no identifiable reason. These assumptions do not have any scientific proof and are based on the examiner's feeling, and incorrectly imply that reactive depression does not require treatment.

Yet, one of you can easily question the need for medications for someone whose depression or sadness can be "explained." For example, it may sound unreasonable to treat someone who is going through grief. But, what if they are predisposed or have a history and the loss precipitates an episode of depression? In fact, stress is a very common risk factor for depression. It is, however, at times difficult to differentiate a depression that is a mood state to depression as a disease, presenting a clinical dilemma.

The clinical decision to treat depression or any condition is based on risks and benefits. Considering the safety of antidepressants, I think, it is reasonable to treat individuals even when their presentation is not

---

3 Ziprasidone is weight neutral, meaning it does not cause heavy weight gain. Ziprasidone was introduced in the US at the time when antipsychotics that cause severe weight gain including olanzapine, quetiapine and risperidone were used heavily. It appears that, due to QT prolongation and death scare, it was not used as frequently as the others. Lack of sedation, twice a day dosing, and the quirky need to take this medication with food (ziprasidone does not get absorbed well on an empty stomach) did not help either.

convincing. However, some patients may resist, feeling that the label of mental illness is stigmatizing and demoralizing. On the other hand, it makes no sense to withhold the medications from someone who may have a chance of benefiting from them, whether it is endogenous, reactive or whatever.

Untreated depression can affect the individual in more ways than their mood. For example, untreated depression in a patient with myocardial infarction doubles the odds of post infarction death. Depression is as serious, if not more serious, as high cholesterol in the morbidity and mortality of heart diseases. Patient attitudes may be a major barrier for treatment. They might say that they are just having a bad day and will get better or they can tough it out. They may choose some natural treatment that they think is harmless and even downing the sorrow with a bottle sound reasonable option. For some, it may be a tougher pill to swallow if you tell them that they need to take a medication for a possible mental illness.

Considering all this, it is a good idea to treat or recommend antidepressants when you are in doubt. However, it may be easier to convince patients to take an anti-cholesterol medication to treat an asymptomatic disease than to convince them to take a pill for a very painful and uncomfortable illness such as depression. Personally, I always recommend my colleagues to treat patients with an SSRI when they suspect depression. At times, patients may be more accepting to take an antidepressant prescribed by a cardiologist or an internist than to follow up on their advice to see a psychiatrist. Patients need to be reassured, both clinicians and patients should have an open mind and make the decision together.

Choosing an Antidepressant

Selective Serotonin Reuptake Inhibitors (SSRIs)

SSRIs are popular first choice of antidepressants and are widely prescribed by primary care physicians and non-psychiatrists because of their high safety profile. SSRIs include fluoxetine (Prozac), sertraline (Zoloft), paroxetine (Paxil), citalopram (Celexa) and escitalopram (Lexapro), an isomer of citalopram and the recent one vortioxetine (Brintellix). Citalopram has gained favored status due to the lower side effect profile. SSRIs are believed to work by increasing the availability of serotonin in the synapse. SSRIs are generally very efficacious and there seems to be no convincing differences between them in terms of efficacy.

Common side effects of SSRIs include GI effects such as nausea vomiting and diarrhea, insomnia, hypersomnia, restlessness (akathisia), and headaches. These are more common in the first few days of treatment and generally subside after the first week. It is prudent to start patients at half or quarter pill and increase the dose over a few days to avoid or minimize these side effects. The patients are frequently advised to take a quarter pill for two or four days, half pill for another two or four days and then the whole pill. Patients with high levels of anxiety tend to struggle with side effects and hesitate to start or build up the dosing. This is especially true when they have restlessness. They need a lot of reassurance.

Sexual side effects are common in SSRIs but can occur with almost any antidepressant except bupropion. Although anorgasmia or inability to reach orgasm is described as the classic side effect of SSRIs, patients report problems with all aspects of sex, including loss of libido, interest, problems with erection or ejaculation. While some men prefer the delay in the orgasm as a tool for prolongation of performance, anorgasmia can be very annoying. Dapoxetine, a short acting SSRI is approved in some countries for premature ejaculation. These sexual side effects are common, and may lead to patients wanting to stop the medication. Sometimes reassurance and patience might help as these side effects may improve or disappear over time. A reduction in dosage or drug holidays (skipping the medicine on the days of sex or taking the pill after sex[4]) may help. Sometimes they may require a change of medication to bupropion. An evaluation of sexual health may help, and some patients may benefit with phosphodiesterase inhibitors such as sildenafil (Viagra).

SSRIs can rarely cause extrapyramidal side effects and falls in the elderly. SSRIs are sometimes used to treat migraines, but they may also cause or worsen migraines. Patients frequently complain of weight gain on SSIRs but weight loss is also common.

Serotonin Syndrome

This is a rare side effect that results from excessive serotonin in the brain. This may result from the use of SSRIs, especially in combination with other drugs that cause an increase in serotonin in the brain, such as MAO inhibitors. High doses of SSRIs in combination with other antidepressants, triptans, tramadol and linezolid, an antibiotic that acts like an MAOI should be avoided. Serotonin syndrome is characterized by high blood pressure and the symptoms may include abdominal pain, diarrhea, excessive sweating, flushing, and myoclonus. Rhabdomyolysis, hyperthermia, renal failure, and shock may result in death. Switching between SSRIs and MAOIs should be done carefully to avoid such drug interaction. It is recommended that 5 half-lives (2 to 6 weeks) elapse between them.

---

4 One of my patients quipped "Can you write that (take after sex) in the script doc?" and added "can I take it three times a day?"

Discontinuation Syndrome

Patients who abruptly stop SSRIs, especially the ones with shorter half-life, experience significant withdrawal symptoms that may look like a flu. Patients report headache, nausea, chills and body aches along with an uncomfortable dizziness or lightheadedness. Some experience paresthesias that feel like painful electric shocks. This could be a very disabling and unsettling experience for some patients. To avoid these side effects, the medication should be tapered over a few weeks before stopping. Patients must be warned about withdrawal and be careful to avoid stopping abruptly.

Serotonin Norepinephrine Reuptake Inhibitors (SNRIs)

SNRIs are generally second choice medications and they may have a slight edge over SSRIs in terms of efficacy. Venlafaxine (Effexor) and duloxetine (Cymbalta) are the two available drugs. The dosing of these medications is a bit more complex than the SSRIs which sometimes may dampen the enthusiasm as the first choice. Venlafaxine is started at 25 mg or 37.5 mg twice a day and increased to 225 mg a day. Occasionally patients may need up to 375 mg. The long acting form of venlafaxine is started at 75 mg a day and can be increased to 225 mg or 375 mg if needed. Duloxetine is started at 20 or 30 mg and a typical maintenance dose is 60 mg. The maximum recommended is 120 mg.

These are the drugs of choice for patients who do not respond to SSRIs. In addition, venlafaxine and duloxetine are shown to help with neuropathic pain and is favored among patients who may have chronic pain. The side effects and withdrawal are very similar to SSRIs except the fact that SNRIs have a tendency to increase the blood pressure. Desvenlafaxine (Pristiq) is the active metabolite of venlafaxine and is essentially the same as venlafaxine. Desvenlafaxine is effective at 50-100 mg a day.

Tricyclic Antidepressants

Tricyclic antidepressants (TCAs) include amitriptyline, nortriptyline, protriptyline, imipramine, desipramine, doxepin and trimipramine. These are older medications, some of which were introduced in the 60s. TCAs are as effective as SSRIs or other medications and they were very popular until the introduction of SSRIs in the 90s. Annoying side effects such as dry mouth and constipation and complex dosing has pushed them behind the SSRIs and SNRIs. Sometimes they are preferred for the sedation and are frequently used in pain clinics as they provide relief from neuropathic pain.

TCAs can cause serious cardiac side effects including tachycardia, orthostatic hypotension, QT prolongation and arrhythmias. Pretreatment ECGs are recommended for people over 50 and those with cardiac history. Sexual side effects and weight gain can also happen with TCAs. Anticholinergic side effects include dry mouth, constipation, urinary hesitancy, difficulty to focus in near vision, and memory impairment. TCAs should be avoided in people with glaucoma, enlarged prostate or dementia. In general, this is not a desirable medication in the elderly or medically unstable, who may experience falls due to sedation or orthostatic hypotension. TCAs are only rarely used these days and are used only when SSRIs and SNRIs fail, but they are popular among pain specialists due to the benefit in neuropathic pain.

Monoamine Oxidase Inhibitors (MAOIs)

MAOIs are also old medications introduced in the 1960s for depression. These were accidentally discovered when iproniazid (isoniazid before that), an anti-tuberculosis medication was noted to elevate the spirits of TB patients. Iproniazid was found to inhibit the enzyme Monoamine Oxidase (MAO). Monoamine oxidase catalyzes monoamines (histamine, dopamine, epinephrine and norepinephrine) and blocking the MAO, leads to a net increase of the monoamines of interest in the brain, which in turn is believed to help with depression. Thus, was born the "Monoamine Theory of Depression." Introduction of MAOI along with the detailed studies of chlorpromazine in schizophrenia heralded the birth of psychopharmacology. MAOIs were popular in the 60s and 70s but fell out of favor because of the dietary restrictions to avoid hypertensive crisis.

Monoamine oxidase was first named as tyramine oxidase by its discoverer, Mary Bernheim, because MAO metabolizes tyramine in the liver. Tyramine is a sympathomimetic drug that increases blood pressure by releasing catecholamines such as epinephrine and norepinephrine peripherally. Tyramine is found in cured, fermented, or spoiled food including a variety of cheeses, cured meats, beer, pickles, kimchi, and so on. MAO metabolizes the dietary tyramine in the liver, saving us from high blood pressure. When someone is taking MAOIs, ingested tyrosine goes unchecked, causing the hypertensive crisis, which can be life threatening, the reason why patients taking MAOI should consume tyramine free diet.

MAOIs include phenelzine, tranylcypromine, isocarboxazid, moclobemide and selegiline. Selegiline is a MAO-B inhibitor and so it has less danger of hypertensive crisis (less, but not nonexistent as MAO-B also metabolizes tyramine). It is available as a patch and so it avoids the first pass in the liver, thus reducing the chance of hypertensive crisis further. Selegiline at the lower dose of 6 mg patch does not require

MAOI diet, but at the higher dose of 9 or 12 mg one needs to follow the dietary restrictions. There is a group of "reversible" MAO-A inhibitors that do not have the tyramine related hypertensive crisis. They are reversible because they are displaced from the MAO-A in the presence of tyramine, and so, the normal metabolism of tyramine is not blocked. Moclobemide, minaprine and caroxazone are some of the reversible MAOI inhibitors available outside of America.

MAOIs are used infrequently for cases of drug resistant depression. There is some evidence that MAOIs may help in atypical depression (irritability, mood reactivity, weight gain and hypersomnia). They are also found to be useful in a variety of anxiety disorders.

Other Antidepressants

Other antidepressants include bupropion (Wellbutrin) or mirtazapine (Remeron), trazodone and nefazodone. Bupropion is structurally related to stimulants and has stimulant properties. It behaves a bit differently compared to other antidepressants. Because of its mild stimulant property, it helps patients with low energy or those who exhibit hypersomnia. It may be weight neutral or help lose weight. It does not have sexual side effects like SSRIs or SNRIs. It may not be as effective as others for patients with high anxiety or anxiety disorders. Bupropion needs to be started at 75 or 150 mg and increased to around 300 for efficacy. The drug was briefly withdrawn after its introduction in the 80s because of seizures, but seizures are rare at doses below 450. Bupropion should not be used among patients with seizures or history of epilepsy. Caution also must be entertained among patients who are drinking heavily or going through alcohol or sedative withdrawals. Bupropion suppresses cravings for nicotine and works well for people who want to quit smoking.

Mirtazapine is a tetracyclic antidepressant with sedation as a prominent side effect. It is an analog of another old tetracyclic antidepressant mianserin. It is not a reuptake inhibitor and is believed to work through adrenergic receptor and may influence serotonergic system indirectly. Trazodone is an antidepressant with sedation as a major side effect, but it is rarely used for depression but widely used as a sedative. Trazodone can cause or contribute to cardiac arrhythmias. Trazodone is used at 25 mg to 100 or 200 mg for sleep and may be effective as an antidepressant at 150 to 400 mg a day. Priapism is a possible side effect of trazodone. Nefazodone is similar to trazodone in structure and side effects. It is pulled off of the US market because of rare hepatotoxicity.

Psychopharmacology

Antidepressants		
Medication (Brand Name)	Usual Dose (mg)	Half-Life (Hours)
SSRIs		
Fluoxetine (Prozac)	20-60	96-144
Sertraline (Zoloft)	50-200	22-36
Paroxetine (Paxil)	20-50	24
Citalopram (Celexa)	20-40	36
Escitalopram (Lexapro)	5-20	30
Vortioxetine (Brintellix)	5-20	66
SNRIs		
Venlafaxine (Effexor)	75-375	4-7
Duloxetine (Cymbalta)	60	8-17
TCAs		
Medication (Brand Name)	Usual Dose (mg)	Half-Life (Hours)
Amitriptyline (Elavil)	75-150	9-25
Nortriptyline (Allegron)	75-100	36
Protriptyline (Vivactil)	15-40	54-92
Imipramine (Tofranil)	75-200	19
Desipramine (Norpramin)	100-200	21-125
Doxepin (Sinepin)	25-300	33-80
Trimipramine (Surmonti)	50-75	23
MAOIs		
Phenelzine (Nardil)	15-45	11-12
Tranylcypromine (Parnate)	20-30	2
Isocarboxazid (Marplan)	10-20	36
Moclobemide (Manerix)	150-600	2-4

Antidepressants		
Selegiline (Eldepryl, Emsam)	6-12	10 (oral), 18-25 (transdermal)
Others		
Bupropion (Wellbutrin)	200-450	12-30
Mirtazapine (Remeron)	15-45	20-40
Trazodone (Oleptro)	150-300	5-13
Nefazodone (Serzone)	200-600	2-4

Mood Stabilizers

The term mood stabilizer is frequently misunderstood. People wrongly attribute this term to a presumed technique by which the medication stabilizes an unstable mood, like fixing the mood swings of day to day life, or calming down the angry, restless, wavering mind. Mood stabilizers help patient with bipolar illness by treating or preventing manic and depressive episodes. Bipolar patients typically get these episodes of depression and mania that last weeks or months and occur over a period of years. They "stabilize" the mood over the years or hopefully during the lifetime of the patient by preventing manic or depressive episodes. The analogies used in the clinic to explain to the patients such as cruise control or thermostat are also misleading because the time line and the mechanism are not similar.

Treatment of bipolar disorder is a challenge. An accurate diagnosis and assessment of the clinical status is essential. Possibly due to the over-diagnosis and excessive mindless use of the term bipolar disorder, the utility of the bipolar disorder diagnosis in the clinical setting has almost lost its meaning. Patients with personality disorders such as borderline personality disorder are frequently diagnosed with bipolar and are even treated like bipolar. It is also common to see patients carrying the diagnosis of bipolar disorder and never been medicated with a mood stabilizer. Often the diagnosis is used and made with low conviction and patients carry them with no adequate knowledge.

Mood stabilizer is the mainstay of the treatment of bipolar disorder. Once the diagnosis is established (again, I cannot overemphasize the need for an affirmative diagnosis. Patients without a manic or hypomanic episode - which is clearly an episode of abnormal and pathological happiness may not be diagnosed with bipolar.), the patients need to be placed on a mood stabilizer. They are required in the acute phases of mania, and depression, as well as for continuation and maintenance treatments. Lithium, valproic acid, carbamazepine, oxcarbazepine, and lamotrigine are proven to help.

Treating a patient with bipolar illness is complex and varies widely depending upon the clinical situation. If a patient presents with mania and is drug naïve, or relapsed after stopping the medication, they need to be started on a mood stabilizer and an antipsychotic. This is also true if they present with mania and psychosis or mixed episode with or without psychosis. If they are already on medications, levels need to be checked and a switch to another antipsychotic may be necessary. If they are taking antidepressants, it needs to be stopped when they are manic. Agitation and hyperactivity may be controlled by benzodiazepines.

If a known or suspected bipolar patient presents with an acute episode of depression, they need to be started on mood stabilizer and an antidepressant. If they are already on medication, the level needs to be checked and dose adjusted. Antidepressant can be switched or augmented with a second antidepressant or a second-generation antipsychotic. Thyroid function needs to be checked because even subclinical hypothyroidism can influence bipolar significantly, causing depression and rapid cycling. Augmentation with thyroid hormone is also a possibility. If the patient is psychotic, an antipsychotic is needed. ECT may be considered in severely ill patients. One must exercise caution because treatment with antidepressants may lead to precipitation of mania.

As the patients improve from the acute illness, they may not need all the medications for the maintenance phase. Antidepressants can be stopped when the depression gets better, and antipsychotics can be stopped when the mania and psychosis improve. Benzodiazepines used for agitation should also be stopped because of the addiction potential. It is ideal for patients to take minimal medications as they go into maintenance phase. Ideally, they could stay on the chosen mood stabilizer alone without the antidepressants or antipsychotics that were used in the acute phase, but this may not happen often. The goal in the maintenance phase is relapse prevention and the mainstay of treatment is a mood stabilizer. However, some patients may need long term use of antidepressants or antipsychotics. It is important to remember to evaluate and reevaluate the patient's clinical situation and medication every visit. Mood stabilizers include lithium, valproic acid, carbamazepine, lamotrigine and oxcarbazepine.

Lithium Carbonate

Lithium carbonate is a salt and it is often referred to as lithium, but lithium is an alkali mineral which is unstable in the free form and is generally available as a salt. Lithium chloride was once used as a salt substitute but was stopped due to side effects and toxicity. The starting dose of lithium (any mention of lithium in this book refers to the lithium carbonate salt sold as a medicine) is typically 300 mg and it can be raised quickly to 900 or 1200 in acute settings. The treatment of lithium is based on the blood level which should be 0.8 to 1.2mmol/L in acute stages and 0.4 to 0.8 for maintenance. The lithium level is tested at its trough, ideally measured 8 hours after the last dose.

Before starting someone on lithium, basic labs to establish kidney and thyroid functions are required. An ECG will also be necessary to establish baseline. They would test the level first thing in the morning before the morning dose. Lithium has a narrow therapeutic window. It is efficacious between 0.8 meq to 1.2 meq per liter. Above 1.5 meq, it is toxic and below 0.4 meq it is non-therapeutic. Levels above 2.0 meq can cause life threatening side effects including cardiac arrhythmias, seizures, coma and neurological damage. These patients may need dialysis. The levels between 0.4 and 0.8 are often sufficient for maintenance and relapse prevention. However, patients who have rapid cycling bipolar (4 episodes in a year) may need to stay at the higher dose.

The immediate side effects of lithium are similar to high salt intake including polydipsia (thirst), polyuria, fluid retention, weight gain and edema. Some patients report sedation, lethargy, impaired coordination, memory problems and confusion. Distinct fine tremor at the fingertips is a sign of high blood level. GI side effects such as nausea and diarrhea are also common. Hair loss, acne, and benign leukocytosis can also occur.

Lithium can cause hypothyroidism after using it for a year or longer. Long term use, for more than 10 years or so can cause changes in the kidney. It is suspected that long term lithium use can cause damage to the kidneys and may cause renal failure, although a direct relationship is debated. Lithium exposure during the pregnancy, especially in the first 10 weeks, has a slight increase in the occurrence of cardiac abnormalities in babies including Epstein's anomaly (an abnormality of the tricuspid valve between the right atrium and right ventricle) and other congenital cardiac defects.

Valproic Acid

Valproic acid is a weak organic acid with valproate as its conjugate base. Sodium valproate is its salt and a combination of sodium valproate and valproic acid is called divalproex sodium. All three formulations; sodium valproate, valproic acid and divalproex sodium are used as antiepileptics and for bipolar disorder.

Valproate is started at the dose of 20-30 mg per kilogram of body weight a day or lower. 250 mg twice a day or 500 mg twice a day is a good starting dose depending upon the acuity of the situation. An average adult may need about 1000 to 2000 mg per day, but some physicians and neurologists push the dose upwards depending upon the clinical situation and side effects. The dose is titrated with a target blood level of 50 to 125 mg/ml. The common side effects include GI effects such as nausea, vomiting, dyspepsia. Sedation is a common side effect that is generally tolerated well. Weight gain and hair loss can be annoying and at times and become the reason to stop the medication. Tremor, leukopenia and thrombocytopenia may occur. Benign increase in transaminase can occur but caution must be exercised in patients with liver problems such as heavy drinkers for whom valproate can be hepatotoxic. Higher incidence of polycystic ovarian syndrome has been found among women who take valproate for epilepsy. Valproate can cause rare, idiosyncratic and potentially life-threatening side effects including liver failure, agranulocytosis, like in clozapine and hemorrhagic pancreatitis.

The major advantage of valproate over lithium is that valproate has a larger therapeutic window. Neurologists often use very high doses. In case of bipolar patients, the therapeutic blood level ranges from 50 to 125 mcg/ml which allows a highly variable dosing. Often, in the clinical setting, clinicians see a lot of room to push the dose up if needed.

Carbamazepine

Carbamazepine is also an antiepileptic medication used for bipolar illness. It is not as well studied as lithium or valproate, but it is believed to be equally effective but is not as popular. Clinically it is chosen when lithium and valproate fail. In recent days, lamotrigine seems to be favored by the clinicians, at least as much as lithium pushing carbamazepine further behind.

The therapeutic dose ranges from 200 mg a day to 1800 mg a day. The dose needs to be started low and moved up slowly. Depending upon the setting (inpatient vs. outpatient) 200 mg once or twice a day and rarely three times a day may be started and raised by 200 a day or a week. The dose is increased based on the clinical improvement, blood level or emergence of side effects. Common side effects include diplopia, fatigue, nausea and ataxia. These may be pronounced when there is a rapid increase in the dosage. Carbamazepine can be toxic and life threatening at 6g. Toxicity or overdose may result in irritability, stupor or coma. Signs of toxicity include, ophthalmoplegia, nystagmus, and EPS. Arrhythmias, seizures and respiratory suppression may also result.

Patients with seizure are maintained at blood level between 4-12 mcg/ml. There is no clear guideline for bipolar, but this is generally used as the target level. Blood level should be obtained in the morning before the AM dose and after at least a week of usage.

Carbamazepine may cause some rare but life-threatening side effects including thrombocytopenia, agranulocytosis, aplastic anemia, pancreatitis, liver failure and exfoliative dermatitis (Stevens-Johnson syndrome) and patients must be educated about this. Like in valproate and lithium, a good baseline physical and lab status needs to be established. CBC, electrolytes and liver function tests should be obtained at baseline and every two weeks until the dose is stable. After the initial period these tests need to be repeated every three months or more frequently if there is any lab abnormality. Carbamazepine is a strong inducer of cytochrome P-450, and it can lead to quicker metabolism and so a reduced level of some drugs including warfarin, lamotrigine, phenytoin, theophylline as well as a number of antipsychotics and antidepressants. Some drugs including fluoxetine, fluvoxamine, cimetidine, and some antibiotics like erythromycin and calcium channel blockers block P-450 and so increase the level of carbamazepine.

Lamotrigine

Lamotrigine (Lamictal) has gained popularity for bipolar illness, especially as a maintenance medication because of the relatively low side effect profile and the ease of monitoring (no need for blood levels or serious hematological side effects compared to other medications). The drug has a serious side effect of a skin rash and Stevens-Johnson syndrome, especially when the dose is titrated quickly. It should be started at 25 mg for the first week or two and increase by 25 mg per week. After 4 weeks on the medication, it can be increased by 50 mg per week. Common side effects include headache, dry mouth, and nausea. Concurrent use of valproate will increase the blood level of lamotrigine and so it should be used at half the dose. Concurrent use of carbamazepine would decrease the level of lamotrigine and so the dose needs to be adjusted up. Patients seem to benefit from 100 mg to 200 mg a day. Lamotrigine is seen as a first line medication for bipolar depression and bipolar maintenance treatment but not as much in acute mania. However, the utility of lamotrigine as a viable alternative to lithium is currently fairly well established. Stopping lamotrigine should also follow similar titer. A quick stoppage may lead to confusion and delirium.

Oxcarbazepine (Trileptal)

Oxcarbazepine is a derivative of carbamazepine, believed to have fewer side effects and it is a weaker inducer of liver enzymes. Although it is not well studied, there is adequate support for its utility in bipolar disorder. It is started at 300 mg twice a day and the maximum dose is 1200 mg per day. No need for a blood level.

Other medications

Second generation antipsychotics are sometimes used alone or together with mood stabilizers in bipolar disorder. Antipsychotics alone or in combination help with mania in the acute setting and may help with depression as an augmenting agent. Other drugs including benzodiazepines such as lorazepam and clonazepam, may help with mania at least by helping with agitation. Some other drugs including calcium channel blockers such as verapamil, zonisamide, acamprosate, omega 3 fatty acids have been reported effective by small studies, but the results are inconclusive. ECT is frequently used in intractable depression and at times in severe mania or mixed episodes. Rare medications and ECT are used for drug resistant patients and used only by the specialists in this disorder.

Anxiolytics

Benzodiazepines such as alprazolam (Xanax), lorazepam (Ativan) or clonazepam (Klonopin) constitute the most widely used anxiolytics. They work on the GABA receptor and almost all of these drugs behave in the same manner and share the side effects and addiction potential. The use of these drugs is discussed elsewhere in the context of therapeutic utility and addiction.

In general, benzodiazepines are very effective in the short term, but patients can easily become dependent and addicted to it. For some patients the benefit of anxiety reduction may lessen or disappear on long term use and they may be taking this to prevent breakthrough anxiety or withdrawal anxiety. It is generally recommended not to prescribe these beyond 2 weeks. Some patients may take a low dose of benzodiazepines for a long time to control anxiety. Any patient who takes more than 3 mg equivalent of lorazepam should be considered dependent and an intervention may be referred. Commonly used benzodiazepines are listed in the table.

Anxiolytics		
Medication (brand name)	Usual dose (Mg)	Half-life (hours)
Alprazolam (Xanax)	0.25 to 2	6-20
Bromazepam (Lectopam)	1.5 to 3	11-22

Anxiolytics		
Chlordiazepoxide (Librium)	5 to 10	5-30
Clonazepam (Klonopin)	0.5 to 1	18-39
Clorazepate (Tranxene)	3.75 to 22.5	40-50
Diazepam (Valium)	5 to 10 mg	20-50
Flurazepam (Dalmane)	15 or 30	<1
Lorazepam (Ativan)	0,5 to 1	10-20
Oxazepam (Serax)	15 or 30	3-21
Temazepam (Restoril)	7.5 to 30	10-20
Triazolam (Halcion)	0.125 to 0.25	1.6-5.5
Midazolam (Versed)	1-2.5 mg Intravenously	1-4

Barbiturates are used at times for anxiety and for benzodiazepine withdrawal. They are not commonly used due to the addiction potential. Non-sedating anti-anxiety medications such as Beta blockers (propranolol) and antihistamines hydroxyzine (Atarax and Vistaril) are non-addictive and are generally effective. Patients, especially those who like benzodiazepines do not prefer these.

Note: Sleep medications and stimulants are discussed in the chapters of insomnia and ADHD.

Chapter 18

Psychotherapy

Psychotherapy is the science of using psychological techniques to change or improve behavior, thought or emotion. Talk therapy, as it is referred by some, can be a powerful tool to help someone who is going through a tough time. Simple moral support, listening ear or an offer of an alternative perspective can change the mood and outlook of someone who is stressed or sad. Grief counseling, Alcoholics Anonymous, and support groups are some excellent examples of how talk therapy can be lifesaving.

However, there is a lot of skepticism for psychotherapy as a treatment modality. It is very difficult to study a psychotherapeutic technique using randomized, double blind, placebo-controlled clinical trials to prove its utility. Psychotherapy is subjective and so bias is a major issue. In addition, there are just too many variables to control. Yet, there are several studies that have shown the benefits of psychotherapy such as CBT or DBT. In this section all non-psychopharmacological modalities are discussed in brief.

Psychoanalysis

As it is discussed in the chapter psychology, psychoanalysis as a therapeutic technique is not practical, lacks any kind of scientific validity and seems to be a thing of a select few who choose to believe its utility as a treatment technique. Only a few select "patients" who are not severely mentally ill, not addicted to substances, psychologically and intellectually sophisticated, are considered eligible for psychoanalysis. These patients are supposed to be bothered by some kind of long-standing internal conflict, which the patient is not actually aware of because consciously uncomfortable desires of the id, are supposedly repressed into the unknown subconscious. As these are unknown to the patient, he or she cannot express it but, the analyst figures them out from a technique called free association, where the so called patient lies on a couch and speaks what comes to his or her mind without censor. This free association reveals itself in some sort of tension between the analyst and analysand by a mechanism called neurosis which is understood by the analyst who "awakens" the patient from the deep misery caused by the deep, unknown conflict. These are done by 3 to 5 sessions per week for 3 to 5 years.

Psychoanalytic Psychotherapy

Psychoanalytic psychotherapy is a shorter (one to three sessions per week for one to 6 years!) and less comprehensive form of therapeutic technique based on the principles of psychoanalysis. Here, the focus can be one or two symptoms and one or two related internal conflicts. The same method of free association and identification of transference neurosis are applied. It is believed that patients develop transference neurosis towards the analyst based on their infantile neurosis or hidden conflicts. The analyst's role is to identify and recognize such a neurosis, and associated resistance to change, because the infantile conflict is uncomfortable and hidden, and is rekindled by the relationship with the therapist. For example, if the patient had a sexual attraction towards one of her parents (which happens to be the nidus for the conflict) and that comes up in the process of analysis as a similar sexual attraction towards the older therapist, which makes her uncomfortable. The analyst also needs to be aware of the countertransference that develops during the sessions because of his or her own repressed conflicts from the past. Analysts typically are required to undergo psychoanalysis themselves.

There are several other therapies and therapeutic techniques based on psychoanalytic principles including insight-oriented psychotherapy, supportive psychotherapy, interpersonal psychotherapy and so on. These techniques are based on the psychoanalytic principles in some form or other. Since Freud, several other psychoanalysts including his daughter Anna Freud came up with variations of the psychoanalytic theory and techniques. A discussion of these is beyond the scope of this book.

Crisis Intervention

Crisis intervention in the conventional sense means when the patient is in a psychological crisis, he or she is seen in a therapy setting to address and manage the crisis. Over the years, crisis intervention has become more medical and is integrated in the emergency rooms. Most of the patients seen in crisis are psychotic or suicidal. They may need support, reassurance, safety and direction along with medications and even brief hospitalization. It is in general, good to remember that benzodiazepines like lorazepam are very helpful when the patient is agitated or anxious.

Group Therapy

The main idea or principle in group therapy is support. Group therapy is very effective in chronic medical illnesses such as end stage cancer, but underutilized. Patients with similar problems gather support from fellow sufferers in a manner that cannot be replicated in any other setting. The way they identify, feel loved, and supported by each other cannot be expected from family members, friends and certainly not from a therapist unless they are also going through the same thing. This is one of the reasons why people who suffer catastrophes as a group form a significant bond. Support groups such as Alcoholics Anonymous, family support groups, victims' groups and so on follow the same principle. A typical group consists of 5 to 12 people with one moderator or therapist. A therapist can be a trained professional like a psychologist, or a recovering patient trained or experienced in group therapy techniques. The role of the therapist is to enable an active discussion, encourage participation, avoid conflicts, and maintain order. Psychoeducation applied in a group setting is a fairly effective tool.

Cognitive Behavioral Therapy

Cognitive therapy and behavioral therapy are sometimes discussed as different modalities of treatment. There is difference in the concept and techniques of cognitive therapy and behavioral therapy, but they overlap and complement each other. A combination of cognitive techniques and behavioral techniques are often used, and these are based on the learning theories and ideas of Pavlov and BF Skinner (discussed in the psychology chapter).

Unlike psychoanalysis where the basis of a maladaptive behavior is believed to be a hidden conflict, which is brought to the surface through unstructured free associations, CBT is based on tangible and identifiable psychological problems that cause the maladaptive behavior. The thought patterns behind the impaired behavior are either obvious, apparent or easily elicited and explained. These techniques are direct and open, and based on learning theories. These are effectively used in disorders with a component of learning in the psychopathology, such as anxiety disorders or phobias.

Cognitive Therapy

Cognitive therapy was developed by Aaron T Beck at the University of Pennsylvania. Beck revolutionized psychotherapy and made it into a practical, scientific and evidence-based tool that can be taught and learned in a structured manner, leaving nothing for assumptions and interpretations. He developed rating scales and various treatment methods for a number of conditions including depression and anxiety disorders. Beck Institute, now run by his daughter Judith Beck, is a leader in educating cognitive therapy.

Cognitive therapy is most used or applied in depression, although this is modified and applied in other diagnoses, such as anxiety or personality disorders. This approach is based on the idea that maladaptive behavior is based on false or inaccurate cognitions, which can be identified and modified resulting in the improvement of such behavior.

Beck described a cognitive triad where patients with depression may have unrealistic negative opinion of themselves, their environment and their future. The patients may feel, by the influence of their negative cognition, that they are not good, their life is not good, and that they are hopeless about the future. These thoughts are almost always exaggerated, and Beck calls them "automatic thoughts," based on false assumptions. A depressed or anxious person may face a small setback and immediately assume that they are not good for anything, their life is miserable, and their future is hopeless.

His treatment method included four steps including; assessment, cognition, behavior and learning. In assessment, automatic thoughts, and false assumptions are identified and listed for intervention. In cognition, these assumptions are tested or challenged for validity. In the third stage, the patients are prompted to use alternative, reality-based explanations in lieu of the negative thoughts. In learning stage, they use these new behaviors or responses routinely to avoid going deeper into negative thinking.

For example, if a patient says, "Everyone will laugh at me if I give a talk" (or "I have the most miserable life") it is almost always inaccurate (obvious in these examples). If the assumption is questioned, the patients will easily and quickly recognize the exaggeration. Now, they will be asked to tell themselves "it is not going to be that bad if I give a talk" or "I am better than so many people." They need to be helped to learn to counter negative thoughts with positive or realistic thoughts to sustain the behavior.

Quite often, patients are asked to write down their worries and examine the validity of their assumptions in those worries. They are also encouraged to identify things they can control or do something about, and not worry about things that are not in their control. This is simple, logical and effective. This method can be therapeutic for depression and anxiety. Psychotherapy can be an adjunct to medications.

Behavior Therapy

Behavior therapy is based on learning theory and conditioning - both classical Pavlovian conditioning and operant conditioning popularized by BF Skinner[1]. The basic principle of behavioral therapy is desensitization or systematic desensitization. This was developed by Joseph Wolpe, a South African psychologist. The idea is simple and powerful. Let us say we develop a fear of something, for example a fear of dogs, because at some point a dog chased us or bit us. The treatment for this fear is a slow, guided exposure to a (friendly) dog until we lose the fear.

Wolpe recommended relaxation techniques along with the exposure to deal with the fear and anxiety. Yoga, meditation, or deep muscle relaxation are proven techniques of relaxation. Once they practice these relaxation techniques, their core anxiety would go down and they become more ready for the anxiety provoking exposure. The exposure needs to be done slowly and step by step starting with the least threatening stimuli (a little fluffy puppy, a doll or even a picture of a dog to start with) and moving up. The phobia or fear of anything can be addressed by this method. If a patient is afraid of going on bridges or airplanes they can start with a small bridge, and with the help of a therapist or a trusted friend and slowly move up. This needs to be systematic, and the patient needs to persevere until the fear is overcome. The more they avoid, the longer it takes to improve, and the stronger the fear would be. A small dose of anxiety reducing drug like propranolol or benzodiazepine can be used prior to the exposure.

Patients with anxiety often have multiple things that they worry about. They can be asked to make a list of anxiety provoking things and situations and rank them in order from least bothersome to the most bothersome. They will start the exposure therapy with the least anxiety provoking stimulus, master it and then move to the more difficult ones. Once the patient sees improvement, they gain confidence and engage more in the exposure.

An interesting treatment method using exposure therapy is called intentional stuttering strategy. This is essentially stuttering intentionally to treat stuttering! People who stutter are anxious about embarrassing themselves, and when they are anxious, they stutter more. In this treatment method, people are asked to stutter intentionally, often to unsuspecting strangers like store clerks. Because they intentionally stutter, and expect to embarrass themselves, they do not have the fear

---

1 At the height of the Cold War and when behaviorism was very popular new science, some thought that anything - in terms of changing or bending human mind and behavior can be achieved. People believed in brain washing and such and even the CIA was involved in this research. But there is no proof of mind bending, mind control or brainwashing using these techniques.

of embarrassment and are also aware that the stuttering is under their control. Such a feeling of control has the opposite effect of fear. As they lose fear, they become less nervous and slowly stop stuttering.

Aversion therapy is somewhat the opposite of the exposure therapy, where an unwanted behavior is paired with a noxious stimulus (like small electric shocks) to make the behavior disappear. A fluid sensitive pad with a loud bell placed in the bed of bed wetter is a good example of aversion therapy. The kid would wake up in panic when he hears the bell and (hopefully) learn to control the bladder. As you can understand, aversion therapy is controversial and presents an ethical dilemma. But such an approach can be applied in disorders of impulse control, like addiction. Controlled exposure and reaction of alcohol to Antabuse has been used in the past to make the people feel aversive to alcohol but this is not a popular therapeutic method. The opposite of aversion is positive reinforcement, which is a simple reward for good behavior. Positive reinforcement using star charts (one star for good behavior and accumulation of stars would lead to rewards like frequent flier miles) are very useful in children to improve positive behavior.

Dialectical Behavior Therapy

DBT was designed by Marsha Linehan for borderline personality disorder (BPD). It is based on CBT principles and well proven to help patients with BPD. Considering the success in BPD, the DBT technique has also become a popular tool for several other disorders including, anxiety, depression, suicidality, addiction and eating disorders.

Patients with BPD seem to have poor regulation of their cognitive, behavioral, and emotional responses to crises – large and small. For example, even simple disappointments in life can push these patients to suicidal thoughts, self-injurious behavior or even suicide. So, applying the basic idea of CBT – identifying assumptions and challenging them - these patients are trained to be mindful or be aware of their thoughts and emotions and develop skills to address their maladaptive behavior. The training focuses on interpersonal skills, distress tolerance and emotional regulation. The mindfulness technique is based on Buddhist philosophy.

Chapter 19

Evaluation of a Patient with Mental Illness.

Psychiatric evaluation follows similar framework as evaluation of a physical illness. You start off with the presenting complaint and continue with the history of present illness and the rest to collect data supporting a suspected diagnosis and ruling out others. Often, establishing the primary reason for the patient's visit or understanding primary symptoms is the most important, difficult, and challenging aspect of the examination. Without data from a physical exam or labs, the entire diagnostic work up involves talking to the patient and taking elaborate history. Most of us who engage with patients feel and believe that we are very good or good enough to talk to patients and obtain history. However, interviewing technique is an art and science. We can and will get better with training and experience. The following are some basic aspects of interviewing. The goal of the interview or psychiatric examination is to obtain clarity of the patient's presentation.

Establish Rapport

A good rapport is essential to get good history. Patients are generally nervous to talk about their mental health issues. Introduce yourself and ask them to say something about themselves. It is a good idea to get to know the patient first by asking them about their job, interests etc., and show interest in their work or hobbies using follow up questions. This will make them relax and feel reassured. We should make good eye contact, be warm, friendly and caring. Making the patient at ease and making them feel that we are here to listen are important. They need to feel and understand that we care. It is recommended that you let them speak for a few minutes before asking specific questions. This will give an opportunity to make an assessment of patient's ability, attitude, sophistication, willingness and openness that will help us guide through the rest of the interview.

Identify the Chief Complaint

Patient's report of what they are suffering from may vary from an accurate description of their symptoms to vague or general complaints. Even when they say they are depressed; it is important to ask them to characterize or describe what they feel. Patients with mania or psychosis may not give a straightforward answer. Informants might help in such situations. What the patient starts off as a chief complaint may not be the main psychopathology. Patients with anxiety may report "feeling worried" which they may perceive as depression or sadness. Patients with poor insight may not even report a problem. Some patients try to explain why they are sad or worried than what they are suffering from. They need redirection. Once the chief complaint is established, we need to ask leading questions to rule out the differential diagnoses. Questioning should not only help us establish the diagnosis but we should also rule out other causes.

Open-ended, Close-ended and Leading Questions

Open ended questions are the questions that cannot be answered with an "yes" or "no" like, "What happened?" or "Can you explain it?" It is very important to use open ended questions like "What is bothering you?" or "How can I help you?" to start an interview. It is very important to use follow up questions like "What do you mean by depression?" or "Can you explain what you feel?" Following this, you can use more close ended questions like "How bad is the anxiety?" "Does it interfere your day to day activities?" Leading questions or clarifications are appropriate and needed but only after initial exploration of the symptoms. It is difficult to interview patients with psychosis. They may not readily admit or explain their hallucinations or delusions as they do not see them as part of an illness. It is wise to ask them in a nonthreatening, circumspect manner, like "Some of my patients have unusual experiences like hearing voices when no one is speaking. Have you had any experience like that?" or "Do you sometimes think that someone is following you or talking behind your back?" "Have you ever felt that people are talking about you in the TV or media?" In general, leading questions or directional questioning should be used after a good rapport is established.

Sensitive Topics

Do not be hesitant to ask about sensitive topics like sex life or drug use. The questioning should be nonthreatening but can be direct. Always follow up with what the patient says, even if it feels irrelevant. For example, if the patient says "I am so depressed, I am not interested in anything in life," follow up with questions about suicidality. Again, open ended questions like "Have you ever thought that life is not worth living?" as opposed to "Are you thinking about suicide?" is a good beginning. Once the patient answers, then you can follow up with further questioning that are more specific like "Have you thought about suicide?"

Ending

When in doubt, it is a good idea to summarize or rephrase your understanding to the patient so that your assessment is clear. You can rephrase your assessment and understanding and ask the patient to correct if needed. You should ask the patient whether there is anything else they want to add "Is there anything that you think I need to know or did we miss anything?" and ask them whether they have any questions. It is very important to tell them what you think is the problem, inform and explain the diagnosis and treatment plan. Reassure them or be open about the prognosis with a hopeful message of how much the patient will improve. Inform them about side effects of medications and the importance of treatment compliance.

Psychiatric Evaluation

Identification

Age, sex, marital status, occupation and living situation. Also record the informant accompanying the patient and their reliability. In this, occupation and living situation are important. Occupation helps to establish the baseline and level of ability or disability. Living situation, for example, home with the family vs. homelessness makes a difference in the treatment plan. For example, an anxious patient or suicidal patient would need support and care at home. I am not able to come up with a justification to include the race of this patient as I see no clinical utility in that data.

Chief Complaint

Usually this starts with the patient's complaint of his or her symptoms as they report it. It is important to ask them to explain the symptoms as they experience. This not only helps you understand the presenting problem, it helps establish rapport. Patients with poor insight such as schizophrenia may not readily admit to symptoms. Patients with substance use will minimize or deny a problem.

History of Present Illness

Not unlike physical exam, the chief complaint needs to be evaluated for the beginning of the symptoms and its progress over time. In general, the psychiatric symptoms start slowly and patients may not be able to tell you the exact date they started having the symptoms. It is not a bad question to ask "Looking back, when do you think you were symptom free?" Most of the psychiatric diagnoses are based on the history than the presentation. Understanding the baseline and the progression of the illness to the point of disruption to their day to day lives is important. Patients with anxiety typically have anxiety symptoms as children or teens. It is also important to ask for any precipitating event that preceded the onset of symptoms. Life events that may influence the symptoms along with any drug use or medical illness that may have contributed to the onset of symptoms should be examined. Information from the informants will also help, especially when the patient is not sure or unwilling. It is important to keep the questions open ended.

Substance Abuse History

Patients would typically minimize the amount and frequency of use. At times, the way questions are framed influences the answer. Instead of asking "How much do you drink?" asking "What is the maximum you can manage to drink in a day?" will produce a more accurate answer. Similarly, "How many days did you drink in the past week?" brings a better answer than "How often you drink?"

Past Psychiatric History

In this section, ask about previous treatments and episodes. A history of medication use would help in identifying what worked and provide the data on side effects.

Family Psychiatric History

It is important to obtain psychiatric history in the family. This will help in the diagnosis as well as treatment response. For example, a patient presenting with depression who has a family history of bipolar disorder should remind one about the risk of mania.

Medical History

Medical history including allergies and current medications: This is important to obtain the medical history because of the interaction of medical illnesses with psychiatric illness as well as the medication interaction.

Social History

Social support or lack of it impacts many psychiatric illnesses, symptoms and recovery. Social support, including someone who can remind the patient to take the medications would help a lot in the recovery of the patient in addition to psychological support and safety.

Mental Status Examination

This includes a report of patient's appearance, presentation, behavior, speech, thought, cognition and judgment.

Diagnostic Impression

Provisional diagnosis (if appropriate) and differential diagnoses are reported here.

Treatment Plan

This section includes prescription medications and psychotherapy recommendations.

Psychiatric Evaluation
Identification
Chief complaint
History of present illness
Substance abuse history
Past psychiatric history
Family psychiatric history
Medical history
Social history
Mental status examination
Diagnostic impression
Treatment plan

Mental Status Examination

Appearance: appropriateness of clothing and attire are informative of patient's level of functioning.

Attitude: whether the patient is friendly, combative, defensive or resistant.

Motor activity: Patient may be slow in depression or due to sedation, agitated in mania or psychosis and restless or apprehensive with anxiety or akathisia.

Eye contact: Patients with psychosis do not present with a steady eye contact. They seem to not make a connection.

Speech: This is described whether the patient is relevant (answering to the questions), and coherent (making sense in the flow of conversation). A description of volume, tone and rate of speech, whether it is normal, pressured or slowed is included here.

Mood: The answer for "How do you feel or How would you describe your mood?" It is reported verbatim, like "I feel depressed."

Affect: this is the examiner's observation of the patient's mood.

Thought: Thought is reflected in speech. The examiner should note whether patient's thoughts are organized and informative. Disorganized speech or loose associations is characteristic of psychosis. A flight of ideas is characteristic of mania. Delusions are listed here. As mentioned above, patients with psychosis do not readily admit to their unusual beliefs and usually the informant describes them.

Perception: A report of hallucinations is included here.

Cognition: in this section, orientation to time, place, person, memory, attention, and intelligence are assessed. Abstraction and asking the patients to explain meanings of proverbs are generally used in psychiatric examination but their utility in the assessment is questionable.

Judgment and insight: Judgment is their decision making and insight is the level of awareness of their symptoms and suffering.

Mental Status Examination
Appearance
Attitude
Psychomotor activity
Eye contact
Speech
Mood
Affect
Thought
Perception
Cognition
Judgment and insight.

Chapter 20

Miscellaneous Topics

Nature vs. Nurture

This is and will be an ongoing topic of heated discussions and debates among the intellectual elite and the common people alike, especially when it comes to intangible human attributes like honesty, intelligence and attitude. When it comes to obvious physical characteristics like skin color it is easy to observe and believe the influence of nature (genes and inheritance) compared to the influence of environment (race vs. Tan) but when the characteristics are intangible and abstract the debate over nature vs. nurture intensifies. For example, skin color can be seen as more genetic compared to someone's attitude which can be assumed to be mostly if not entirely acquired and so environmental. Height and intelligence may be seen as significantly biological attributes with a good environmental influence. The interplay of nature and nurture is complex and the more we know, it seems that more things are inherited, genetic and biological, at least predominantly.

For example, it may be surprising to know that our ability to learn and master a language is mostly biological and hard wired, probably based on some genes. So, a child born with the right genes resulting in excellent language skills could become a poet but what language he or she becomes an expert in depends upon where he or she grows up. Religious faith is another interesting example because we essentially pick our religion from the parents who raise us but our willingness and ability to question or follow a faith may be more biological.

Mental illness, at least most of them seem to run in families and so are inherited. It is estimated that illnesses like schizophrenia and even our capacity to feel happiness is about 80% dependent on the genes or our biology. It seems that our intellectual and emotional traits and attitudes are biologically determined similar to our height, weight and skin color. But, it is also clear that some strong attributes such as religious faith develop from the environment and so are acquired skills that involve practice and learning like musical talent and athletic ability.

To complicate further, the environmental influence on the biology also gets complex. Some environmental influences like injuries to the brain affecting its development are obvious. Those injuries can be chemical insult such as alcohol or malnutrition during pregnancy or later. However, stress to the mother or the child in terms of neglect or abuse can also alter the biological development of the brain. Physical, chemical and psychological insults can influence and alter the developing brain. It is also to be noted that the same insult or stress may affect individuals differently based on their genetic and biological make up.

Stress, nutrition and drugs or injuries continue to shape the brain of a developing child until age 18 or possibly until age 25 although the effect reduces exponentially. It is recently understood that environmental influences - psychological or chemical - change the way the genes work by turning the genetic switches on and off, a mechanism known as epigenetics. Some believe that epigenetics may answer many complex diseases including mental illnesses. It is important to remember that nature may play a major role in what we are and what kind of illness we get (call it fate or Karma) it is also important to understand the value of nurture. The influence we can exert over our shortcomings by external manipulation with medicine, therapy, learning and training may be limited but are tremendously useful and frequently lead us to a better life, if not life-saving. Designing our nature is a thing of science fiction which may or may not happen.

What is Happiness? or How to Make Yourself Happy?

If you are part of any social group, you would have received some message or a poster telling you how to be happy. You also may have found someone who is obsessed with the idea of making themselves happier (but actually unhappy). Doesn't it make sense that happy people do not worry too much about being happy because they already are?!

In fact, there is only one simple thing that we can all employ to improve our day to day happiness. It is honesty. Honesty in anything and everything in day to day life increases the level of perceived and reported happiness.

Morten L Kringelbach of Oxford defined three components of happiness including 1) Hedonia, the trait or temperament of an individual (or capacity to be happy), which can be biological and genetic. 2) Eudaimania, defined as a fulfilling life (education, marriage, job, wealth etc.), and 3) Engagement, meaning spending our lives doing something (that makes us happier).

Factors that influence happiness in a society or a country include wealth, jobs, personal freedom, transparency and lack of corruption. In addition, a good marriage, intact family, a lot of social support and friends seem to bring happiness.

It is believed that 48% of our happiness is biological, including our genetic make-up and how we are put together. About 40% of it is due to the life situation (wealth, job, relationship) and only 12% is considered to be responsible for the day to day variations - which we can manipulate. While this may be surprising, it is not uncommon to come across people with negative attitude and complaining even when they are comfortable and people who stay happy and positive despite dire circumstances in their lives.

Happiness in the brain uses the same pleasure network (described elsewhere) associated with food, sex and drugs. Various neurochemicals including endocannabinoids, endorphins, dopamine, serotonin, oxytocin, adrenaline and a few others are involved in happiness .

Besides improving life situation and treating mental illnesses like depression, there are a few other things that are essential for a happy life. Having a goal or motivation, not being lazy, setting aside time to reflect on moments of gratitude, altruism, honesty, pursuit of significant life goals, understanding important values in life and the awareness of mortality and consideration of life as a finite and quick one will help. Mindfulness or mentalizing is a technique based on Buddhist philosophy in which one can train to watch his or her thoughts and emotions as they happen and deal with them at the moment. This technique is shown to improve positive thoughts and feelings.

Some things like honesty, humility, generosity, forgiveness are things that our elders and culture repeatedly emphasize for a good life and keep coming again and again in happiness related research. Avoiding mind wandering or not being focused on the task at hand (Matt Killingsworth), slowing down or taking it easy (Carl Honore), having less stuff as possession (Graham Hill and John Lennon) and being grateful to everyone (David Steidnl) are some other ideas proposed by several popular happiness scientists.

The benefits of happy life or even a happy day or a happy moment are enormous. Happy people live longer and obviously happier! They are more productive, friendly and social with a larger network of family and friends. They have better physical and mental health, have stronger and more loving marriages, and intact, caring families.

Miscellaneous Topics

Medical Marijuana

The word Medical Marijuana sounds like an oxymoron because it has not proven to be a medicine by any means and certainly not by the standards of how other medications are proven and approved. It is not prescribed by "regular" doctors and are not dispensed as a medicine in regular pharmacies. But under the medical marijuana law, it is legal to grow, process and sell as a medical product by its own strange clinics and dispensaries. If my writing above sounds defensive, it is because of the changing attitude in the society and my constant struggle with pot smoking patients. At best, the concept of medical marijuana is a political, policy decision of decriminalization and partial legalization and certainly not a new treatment.

The attitude towards marijuana as a medicine is changing drastically around the world, unfortunately in the wrong direction. I am not talking about legalization which is a completely different issue. Legalization of recreational cannabis seems transparent, clear and straightforward. While legalization would continue to uphold the belief that this is a drug used for recreation like alcohol or cocaine, the very term medical marijuana is misleading.

Along with the false perception of marijuana being a medicine, that too a natural and herbal one and so must be safe to consume, and no overdose deaths and so on, this drug is being masqueraded and marketed for the next generation who will see this legalized as a recreational drug soon, which ironically would be a relief, in a quirky manner.

In some ways, this is partial legalization which may not be a major problem as such, but everyone needs to be aware that the emperor does not have clothes when it is sold as a medicine, especially children and teenagers. Marijuana is a drug that is used for recreational purpose. Period. It may have some medicinal properties, but it is not a medicine. People who are terminally ill or even marginally ill who want to use this for any reason can use it if they want to, but it is still not medicine. It is not proven to be superior to what is available out there for nausea, glaucoma, or pain. Still, I do not have a problem if someone wants to use it and if it is legalized.

Cannabis is another drug like alcohol. Nothing more. Nothing less. By the way, alcohol was used as a "medicine" in old days and it does have some medicinal properties (for cough and cold), and a number of cough syrups and mouthwash has alcohol, but I am sure, the idea of medical alcohol or medical margarita sounds funny.

The perception of this being a medicine causes major problems for people like me who are practicing psychiatrists who happen to see an 18-year-old psychotic kid who does not get better because he smokes cannabis heavily. He or she comes and argues that the cannabis they consume is a medicine and is helping them while there is indisputable evidence that cannabis or any street drug that is used heavily and regularly harms people especially those with psychiatric issues.

If the society wants to legalize marijuana or any other drug for recreation, it should be ready to face and deal with the consequences. Availability will increase the incidence of addiction. Addiction and illicit drug use are not going to go away, and some may argue for legalization of all drugs, regulate them and deal with the (increasing number of) addicts. But this is a larger societal policy issue and it is undeniable that legalization will produce more addicts.

However, the idea or medical marijuana is an insult to the intelligence of any rational human being and the way it is implemented is a joke. Doctors with a medical license are prescribing and issuing permits to hundreds of "patients" with all kinds of fake illnesses propagating the tenacious idiots a reason and excuse to light up. I would rather see cannabis next to oregano in the grocery store or in the liquor store than in a doctor's office. At the same time, I believe that there should be valid medical research to investigate in a scientific manner to identify the possible medicinal uses of the herb. Feeling cannot trump science. In the next few decades, most of the world would see legal pot and ironically, it sounds to be a good thing compared to the oxymoronic idea of medical marijuana[1].

---

[1] Of the many interesting conversations and arguments, I had with my patients who smoke chronically (pun intended) some are really interesting and funny.
Marijuana is natural. One mom told me about her 12-year-old son "I don't mind him smoking weed. It is natural, but I don't like him buying in the streets. I don't know what they add in it."
"Well, Poison Ivy is natural. Would you use a soap made by Poison Ivy?"
"Would you be OK, if I, the doctor smoked pot?"
"Actually Doctor, I would rather that you are a pot smoker" "You will understand what we are talking about" - by a 34-year-old lady who starts her days with two joints in the morning.
I smiled and said, "Would you be OK if you take your daughter to the emergency room and the doctor there tell you she would smoke a joint or two before she operates on your kid?"

Glossary

Affect: Observed and expressed emotional behavior is described as affect.
Akinesia: reduction in the voluntary movement.
Alexithymia: is a difficulty in recognizing one's own emotions.
Alogia: Speechlessness or reduced flow of speech.
Ambivalence: Being indecisive or having contradictory ideas. Usually described as a mental state in psychosis.
Amnesia: Pathological loss of memory. Anterograde amnesia is an inability to form new memories and retrograde amnesia is loss of memory of past events.
Amotivation: Lack of motivation as a negative symptom of schizophrenia.
Avolition: Lack of initiative or desire to do something.
Binge drinking: Consuming excessive amounts of alcohol (or drugs or food) in a short amount of time.
Catalepsy: A trancelike state.
Cataplexy: Loss of muscle tone without loss of consciousness. Common in narcolepsy.
Catatonia: Increased muscle tone resulting in rigidity and waxy flexibility.
Circumstantiality: Talking with excessive details surrounding the topic of conversation without coming to the point or losing the point.
Comorbidity: Occurrence of two or more disorders.
Compulsion: A behavior or a thought (hand washing or saying a number) to reduce the anxiety arising from obsessions.
Conditioning: Learning a new behavior or response to a stimulus.
Confabulation: Filling the gaps in knowledge with imagined details to compensate for the lack of memory (in dementia).
Conversion: Referred to the physiological or physical symptoms such as paralysis resulting from a psychological conflict, which is typically uncomfortable for the patient to express.
Coprolalia: Blurting out profanities (in Tourette's syndrome).

Countertransference: A psychoanalytic principle describing the therapist's emotional response to a patient, supposedly based on the therapist's unconscious needs and conflicts.
Defense mechanisms: Used to describe unconscious psychological processes that reduce internal anxiety.
Delusion: A fixed false belief that is out of the patient's cultural norm.
Depersonalization: Feeling that self or the environment is unreal.
Derealization: Feeling detached from one's environment.
Detachment: Interpersonal aloofness.
Disorientation: Lack of awareness or self, others, place and time.
Dystonia: Involuntary and random muscle contraction.
Echolalia: Repeating what one hears.
Echopraxia: Copying action of another person.
Ego: A psychoanalytic principle of the conscious self (as opposed to id, which is subconscious and superego which is the moral aspect of the self)
Ego-dystonic: Symptoms, thought or behavior that are not seen as part of themselves.
Ego-syntonic: Symptoms, thought or behavior that are seen as part of themselves.
Flashback: A symptom of PTSD in which the patient relives or re-experiences the trauma as if it happens now.
Flight of ideas: A symptom of mania where a patient, who is usually pressured in speech and jumps from one topic to another. Usually there is a connection between the topics.
Flooding: A behavioral therapy technique where the patient is exposed to the phobic stimulus intensively.
Free association: A psychoanalytic technique in which the patient (analysand) talks freely about what comes to his or her mind.
Grandiosity: Exaggerated self-worth.
Hypnogogic: Referring to falling asleep.
Hypnopompic: Referring to waking up.
Ideas of reference: Patient's personalized interpretation of common events that they claim are directed towards them.
Incoherence: Speech or thought that is not understandable because it lacks logical connections.
Insight: Awareness of illness, symptoms or behavior.
Introversion: Being shy or asocial (opposite of extroversion).
La belle indifference: A lack of genuine concern for the disability in conversion disorder.

Magical thinking: Imaginary cause and effect (saying a specific number to avert a disaster).
Narcissism: Self-love.
Negative symptoms: of schizophrenia include loss of function.
Neuroleptic Malignant Syndrome: A serious side effect of antipsychotic medications that may be life threatening.
Obsession: A recurrent intrusive thought, image or an impulse that is irrational.
Paranoia: Thinking based on suspicion.
Polydipsia: Excessive thirst.
Pressured speech: Speaking excessively.
Projection: A defense mechanism in which the person attributes his or her problems on to others (unconsciously).
Splitting: Perceiving others as all good or all bad (black and white thinking).
Transference: A psychoanalytic principle of what the patient feels towards the therapist, based on unconscious conflicts.
Waxy flexibility: Increase in muscle tone resulting in joints moving like lead pipe.
Word salad: Extreme form of thought disorder in which the patient utters a bunch of disconnected words.

Bibliography

Abraha, I., Rimland, J. M., Trotta, F. M., Dell'Aquila, G., Cruz-Jentoft, A., Petrovic, M., ... Cherubini, A. (2017, March 1). Systematic review of systematic reviews of non-pharmacological interventions to treat behavioural disturbances in older patients with dementia. the SENATOR-OnTop series. BMJ Open, Vol. 7. https://doi.org/10.1136/bmjopen-2016-012759

Andreasen, N C. (1979). Thought, language, and communication disorders. I. Clinical assessment, definition of terms, and evaluation of their reliability. Archives of General Psychiatry, 36(12), 1315–1321. https://doi.org/10.1001/archpsyc.1979.01780120045006

Andreasen, Nancy C., Nopoulos, P., Schultz, S., Miller, D., Gupta, S., Swayze, V., & Flaum, M. (1994). Positive and negative symptoms of schizophrenia: past, present, and future. Acta Psychiatrica Scandinavica, 90, 51–59. https://doi.org/10.1111/j.1600-0447.1994.tb05891.x

Argiolas, A., & Melis, M. R. (2003). The neurophysiology of the sexual cycle. Journal of Endocrinological Investigation, 26(3 Suppl), 20–22. Retrieved from http://www.ncbi.nlm.nih.gov/pubmed/12834016

Arruda, E. H., & Paun, O. (2017, June 1). Dementia Caregiver Grief and Bereavement: An Integrative Review. Western Journal of Nursing Research, Vol. 39, pp. 825–851. https://doi.org/10.1177/0193945916658881

Asmundson, G. J. G., Taylor, S., & Smits, J. A. J. (2014). Panic disorder and agoraphobia: An overview and commentary on DSM-5 changes. Depression and Anxiety, Vol. 31, pp. 480–486. https://doi.org/10.1002/da.22277

Balaratnasingama, S., & Janca, A. (2015, January 11). Normal personality, personality disorder and psychosis: current views and future perspectives. Current Opinion in Psychiatry, Vol. 28, pp. 30–34.

Ban, T. A. (2007). Fifty years chlorpromazine: A historical perspective. Neuropsychiatric Disease and Treatment, Vol. 3, pp. 495–500.

Brand, B. L. (2012, July). What We Know and What We Need to Learn About the Treatment of Dissociative Disorders. Journal of Trauma and Dissociation, 13(4), 387–396. https://doi.org/10.1080/15299732.2012.672550

Brand, B. L., Sar, V., Stavropoulos, P., Krüger, C., Korzekwa, M., Martínez-Taboas, A., & Middleton, W. (2016). Separating fact from fiction: An empirical examination of six myths about dissociative identity disorder. Harvard Review of Psychiatry, 24(4), 257–270. https://doi.org/10.1097/

Brown, T. A., & Keel, P. K. (2012). Current and emerging directions in the treatment of eating disorders. Substance Abuse : Research and Treatment, 6, 33–61. https://doi.org/10.4137/SART.S7864

Brunello, N., Akiskal, Boyer, P., Gessa, G. L., Howland, R. H., Langer, S. Z., Wessely, S. (1999). Dysthymia: Clinical picture, extent of overlap with chronic fatigue syndrome, neuropharmacological considerations, and new therapeutic vistas. Journal of Affective Disorders, 52(1–3), 275–290. https://doi.org/10.1016/S0165-0327(98)00163-3

Bryant, R. A. (2017). Posttraumatic stress disorder. In The Science of Cognitive Behavioral Therapy (pp. 319–336). https://doi.org/10.1016/B978-0-12-803457-6.00013-1

Butler, A. C., Chapman, J. E., Forman, E. M., & Beck, A. T. (2006). The empirical status of cognitive-behavioral therapy: A review of meta-analyses. Clinical Psychology Review, 26(1), 17–31. https://doi.org/10.1016/j.cpr.2005.07.003

Caligor, E., Levy, K. N., & Yeomans, F. E. (2015, May 1). Narcissistic personality disorder: Diagnostic and clinical challenges. American Journal of Psychiatry, Vol. 172, pp. 415–422. https://doi.org/10.1176/appi.ajp.2014.14060723

Cerbone, A. R. (2017). Introduction: Science, Sexuality, and Psychotherapy: Shifting Paradigms. Journal of Clinical Psychology, 73(8), 926–928. https://doi.org/10.1002/jclp.22506

Chiriţă, A. L., Gheorman, V., Bondari, D., & Rogoveanu, I. (2015). Current understanding of the neurobiology of major depressive disorder. Romanian Journal of Morphology and Embryology, Vol. 56, pp. 651–658. Editura Academiei Romane.

Clemow, D. B., & Walker, D. J. (2014, January 1). The potential for misuse and abuse of medications in ADHD: A review. Postgraduate Medicine, Vol. 126, pp. 64–81. https://doi.org/10.3810/pgm.2014.09.2801

Commonly Abused Drugs Charts | National Institute on Drug Abuse (NIDA). (n.d.). Retrieved October 20, 2019, from https://www.drugabuse.gov/drugs-abuse/commonly-abused-drugs-charts

Cozzi, G., Minute, M., Skabar, A., Pirrone, A., Jaber, M., Neri, E., … Barbi, E. (2017). Somatic symptom disorder was common in children and adolescents attending an emergency department complaining of pain. Acta Paediatrica, International Journal of Paediatrics, 106(4), 586–593. https://doi.org/10.1111/apa.13741

Dimellis, D., Carvalho, A. F., Gonda, X., Fountoulakis, K. N., Vieta, E., & McIntyre, R. S. (2014). Rapid Cycling in Bipolar Disorder. The Journal of Clinical Psychiatry, 75(06), e578–e586. https://doi.org/10.4088/jcp.13r08905

Direkvand-Moghadam, A., Sayehmiri, K., Delpisheh, A., & Satar, K. (2014). Epidemiology of premenstrual syndrome, a systematic review and meta-analysis study. Journal of Clinical and Diagnostic Research, 8(2), 106–109. https://doi.org/10.7860/JCDR/2014/8024.4021

Dispatches from the Freud Wars: Psychoanalysis and Its Passions Retrieved October 20, 2019,

Döpfner, M., Breuer, D., Wille, N., Erhart, M., Ravens-Sieberer, U., & BELLA study group. (2008). How often do children meet ICD-10/DSM-IV criteria of attention deficit-/hyperactivity disorder and hyperkinetic disorder? Parent-based prevalence rates in a national sample--results of the BELLA study. European Child & Adolescent Psychiatry, 17 Suppl 1, 59–70. https://doi.org/10.1007/s00787-008-1007-y

Executive Summary | Surgeon General's Report on Alcohol, Drugs, and Health. (n.d.). Retrieved October 20, 2019, from https://addiction.surgeongeneral.gov/executive-summary

Fawcett, E. J., Fawcett, J. M., & Mazmanian, D. (2016, June 1). A meta-analysis of the worldwide prevalence of pica during pregnancy and the postpartum period. International Journal of Gynecology and Obstetrics, Vol. 133, pp. 277–283. https://doi.org/10.1016/j.ijgo.2015.10.012

Fazel, S., & Danesh, J. (2002). Serious mental disorder in 23000 prisoners: A systematic review of 62 surveys. Lancet, 359(9306), 545–550. https://doi.org/10.1016/S0140-6736(02)07740-1

Flaherty, J. H., Yue, J., & Rudolph, J. L. (2017, August 1). Dissecting Delirium: Phenotypes, Consequences, Screening, Diagnosis, Prevention, Treatment, and Program Implementation. Clinics in Geriatric Medicine, Vol. 33, pp. 393–413. https://doi.org/10.1016/j.cger.2017.03.004

Gelenberg, A. J., Marlene Freeman, C. P., Markowitz, J. C., Rosenbaum, J. F., Thase, M. E., Trivedi, M. H., ... Silbersweig, D. A. (2010). PRACTICE GUIDELINE FOR THE Treatment of Patients With Major Depressive Disorder Third Edition WORK GROUP ON MAJOR DEPRESSIVE DISORDER. Retrieved from http://www.psychiatryonline.com/pracGuide/pracGuideTopic_7.aspx.

Giedd, J. N., Raznahan, A., Alexander-Bloch, A., Schmitt, E., Gogtay, N., & Rapoport, J. L. (2015). Child psychiatry branch of the National Institute of Mental Health longitudinal structural magnetic resonance imaging study of human brain development. Neuropsychopharmacology : Official Publication of the American College of Neuropsychopharmacology, 40(1), 43–49. https://doi.org/10.1038/npp.2014.236

Glenn, A. L., Johnson, A. K., & Raine, A. (2013). Antisocial personality disorder: a current review. Current Psychiatry Reports, 15(12), 427. https://doi.org/10.1007/s11920-013-0427-7

Goldstein, B. I., Birmaher, B., Carlson, G. A., DelBello, M. P., Findling, R. L., Fristad, M., ... Youngstrom, E. A. (2017). The International Society for Bipolar Disorders Task Force report on pediatric bipolar disorder: Knowledge to date and directions for future research. Bipolar Disorders, 19(7), 524–543. https://doi.org/10.1111/bdi.12556

Harrington, B. C., Jimerson, M., Haxton, C., & Jimerson, D. C. (2015). Initial evaluation, diagnosis, and treatment of anorexia nervosa and bulimia nervosa. American Family Physician, 91(1), 46–52.

Hasnain, M., & Vieweg, W. V. R. (2014). QTc interval prolongation and torsade de pointes associated with second-generation antipsychotics and antidepressants: a comprehensive review. CNS Drugs, 28(10), 887–920. https://doi.org/10.1007/s40263-014-0196-9

Hay, P. J., Bacaltchuk, J., & Stefano, S. (2004). Psychotherapy for bulimia nervosa and binging. The Cochrane Database of Systematic Reviews, (3), CD000562. https://doi.org/10.1002/14651858.CD000562.pub2

Healy, D. (2002). The creation of psychopharmacology. Harvard University Press.

Hinshaw, S. P. (2018). Attention Deficit Hyperactivity Disorder (ADHD): Controversy, Developmental Mechanisms, and Multiple Levels of Analysis. Annual Review of Clinical Psychology, 14(1), 291–316. https://doi.org/10.1146/annurev-clinpsy-050817-084917

Hirschtritt, M. E., Bloch, M. H., & Mathews, C. A. (2017, April 4). Obsessive-compulsive disorder advances in diagnosis and treatment. JAMA - Journal of the American Medical Association, Vol. 317, pp. 1358–1367. https://doi.org/10.1001/jama.2017.2200

Hofmann, S. G., Gutner, C. A., & Fang, A. (2012). Social Anxiety Disorder. In Encyclopedia of Human Behavior: Second Edition (pp. 450–455). https://doi.org/10.1016/B978-0-12-375000-6.00330-X

Holden, M., & Kelly, C. (2002). Use of cholinesterase inhibitors in dementia. Advances in Psychiatric Treatment, 8(2), 89–96. https://doi.org/10.1192/apt.8.2.89

Holmes, T. H. (1978). Life situations, emotions, and disease. Psychosomatics, 19(12), 747–754. https://doi.org/10.1016/S0033-3182(78)70891-1

Hurd, M. D., Martorell, P., Delavande, A., Mullen, K. J., & Langa, K. M. (2013). Monetary costs of dementia in the United States. New England Journal of Medicine, 368(14), 1326–1334. https://doi.org/10.1056/NEJMsa1204629

Introductory Textbook of Psychiatry: Donald W. Black / Nancy C. Andreasen: 9789386217899: Amazon.com: Books. (n.d.). Retrieved October 20, 2019, from https://www.amazon.com/Introductory-Textbook-Psychiatry-Black-Andreasen/dp/9386217899

Jordan, A. H., & Litz, B. T. (2014). Prolonged grief disorder: Diagnostic, assessment, and treatment considerations. Professional Psychology: Research and Practice, 45(3), 180–187. https://doi.org/10.1037/a0036836

Kalra, G., Ventriglio, A., & Bhugra, D. (2015, September 3). Sexuality and mental health: Issues and what next? International Review of Psychiatry, Vol. 27, pp. 463–469. https://doi.org/10.3109/09540261.2015.1094032

Kaplan and Sadock's synopsis of psychiatry: Behavioral sciences, clinical psychiatry, 7th ed. - PsycNET. (n.d.). Retrieved October 20, 2019, from https://psycnet.apa.org/record/1994-98050-000

Keshavan, M. S., Giedd, J., Lau, J. Y. F., Lewis, D. A., & Paus, T. (2014). Changes in the adolescent brain and the pathophysiology of psychotic disorders. The Lancet. Psychiatry, 1(7), 549–558. https://doi.org/10.1016/S2215-0366(14)00081-9

Kessler, R. C., Berglund, P., Demler, O., Jin, R., Merikangas, K. R., & Walters, E. E. (2005, June). Lifetime prevalence and age-of-onset distributions of DSM-IV disorders in the national comorbidity survey replication. Archives of General Psychiatry, Vol. 62, pp. 593–602. https://doi.org/10.1001/archpsyc.62.6.593

Kleeblatt, J., Betzler, F., Kilarski, L. L., Bschor, T., & Köhler, S. (2017, May 1). Efficacy of off-label augmentation in unipolar depression: A systematic review of the evidence. European Neuropsychopharmacology, Vol. 27, pp. 423–441. https://doi.org/10.1016/j.euroneuro.2017.03.003

Kringelbach ML, Berridge KC. 2010 Summer; The Neuroscience of Happiness and Pleasure. Soc Res (New York). 77(2):659-678.

Laferton, J. A. C., Stenzel, N. M., Rief, W., Klaus, K., Brähler, E., & Mewes, R. (2017). Screening for DSM-5 Somatic Symptom Disorder: Diagnostic Accuracy of Self-Report Measures Within a Population Sample. Psychosomatic Medicine, 79(9), 974–981. https://doi.org/10.1097/PSY.0000000000000530

Lee, H., Kim, S. S., You, K. S., Park, W., Yang, J. H., Kim, M., & Hayman, L. L. (n.d.). Asian flushing: genetic and sociocultural factors of alcoholism among East asians. Gastroenterology Nursing : The Official Journal of the Society of Gastroenterology Nurses and Associates, 37(5), 327–336. https://doi.org/10.1097/SGA.0000000000000062

Linehan, M M, Comtois, K. A., Murray, A. M., Brown, M. Z., Gallop, R. J., Heard, H. L., ... Lindenboim, N. (2006). Two-year randomized controlled trial and follow-up of dialectical behavior therapy vs therapy by experts for suicidal behaviors and borderline personality disorder.[Erratum appears in Arch Gen Psychiatry. 2007 Dec;64(12):1401]. Archives of General Psychiatry, 63(7), 757–766.

Linehan, Marsha M., Korslund, K. E., Harned, M. S., Gallop, R. J., Lungu, A., Neacsiu, A. D., … Murray-Gregory, A. M. (2015). Dialectical behavior therapy for high suicide risk in individuals with borderline personality disorder: A randomized clinical trial and component analysis. JAMA Psychiatry, 72(5), 475–482. https://doi.org/10.1001/jamapsychiatry.2014.3039

Longo, D. L., James Blair, R. R., Leibenluft, E., & Pine, D. S. (2014). Conduct Disorder and Callous–Unemotional Traits in Youth. Psychopathic Tr a it s. N Engl J Med, 23371(4), 2207–2216. https://doi.org/10.1056/NEJMra1315612

Loureiro-Vieira, S., Costa, V. M., de Lourdes Bastos, M., Carvalho, F., & Capela, J. P. (2017). Methylphenidate effects in the young brain: friend or foe? International Journal of Developmental Neuroscience : The Official Journal of the International Society for Developmental Neuroscience, 60, 34–47. https://doi.org/10.1016/j.ijdevneu.2017.04.002

Love and the Brain | Department of Neurobiology. (n.d.). Retrieved October 20, 2019, from https://neuro.hms.harvard.edu/harvard-mahoney-neuroscience-institute/brain-newsletter/and-brain-series/love-and-brain

Lyssenko, L., Schmahl, C., Bockhacker, L., Vonderlin, R., Bohus, M., & Kleindienst, N. (2018). Dissociation in psychiatric disorders: A meta-analysis of studies using the dissociative experiences scale. American Journal of Psychiatry, 175(1), 37–46. https://doi.org/10.1176/appi.ajp.2017.17010025

MacPhee, E. (2013). Dissociative disorders in medical settings topical collection on complex medical-psychiatric issues. Current Psychiatry Reports, 15(10). https://doi.org/10.1007/s11920-013-0398-8

Malaspina, D., Owen, M. J., Heckers, S., Tandon, R., Bustillo, J., Schultz, S., … Carpenter, W. (2013). Schizoaffective Disorder in the DSM-5. Schizophrenia Research, 150(1), 21–25. https://doi.org/10.1016/j.schres.2013.04.026

McGough, J. J. (2016). Treatment Controversies in Adult ADHD. The American Journal of Psychiatry, 173(10), 960–966. https://doi.org/10.1176/appi.ajp.2016.15091207

Millon, T. (2016). What is a personality disorder? Journal of Personality Disorders, 30(3), 289–306. https://doi.org/10.1521/pedi.2016.30.3.289

Mokhtari, M., & Rajarethinam, R. (2013). Early intervention and the treatment of prodrome in schizophrenia: a review of recent developments. Journal of Psychiatric Practice, 19(5), 375–385. https://doi.org/10.1097/01.pra.0000435036.83426.94

Motta-Mena, N. v., & Puts, D. A. (2017, May 1). Endocrinology of human female sexuality, mating, and reproductive behavior. Hormones and Behavior, Vol. 91, pp. 19–35. https://doi.org/10.1016/j.yhbeh.2016.11.012

Muth, C. C. (2017). Tics and Tourette Syndrome. JAMA, 317(15), 1592. https://doi.org/10.1001/jama.2017.0547

Ng, F., Hallam, K., Lucas, N., & Berk, M. (2007). The role of lamotrigine in the management of bipolar disorder. Neuropsychiatric Disease and Treatment, Vol. 3, pp. 463–474.

Nock, M. K., Kazdin, A. E., Hiripi, E., & Kessler, R. C. (2006). Prevalence, subtypes, and correlates of DSM-IV conduct disorder in the National Comorbidity Survey Replication. Psychological Medicine, 36(5), 699–710. https://doi.org/10.1017/S0033291706007082

Noller, D. T. (2016). Distinguishing disruptive mood dysregulation disorder from pediatric bipolar disorder. Journal of the American Academy of Physician Assistants, 29(6), 25–28. https://doi.org/10.1097/01.JAA.0000483092.35899.a7

O'Connell, B., & Dowling, M. (2014). Dialectical behaviour therapy (DBT) in the treatment of borderline personality disorder. Journal of Psychiatric and Mental Health Nursing, 21(6), 518–525. https://doi.org/10.1111/jpm.12116

O'Hara, M. W., & McCabe, J. E. (2013). Postpartum Depression: Current Status and Future Directions. Annual Review of Clinical Psychology, 9(1), 379–407. https://doi.org/10.1146/annurev-clinpsy-050212-185612

Oliver G. Cameron, M. P. (2007). Understanding Comorbid Depression and Anxiety.

Os, J. van, & Kapur, S. (2012). Seminar SchizophrOs, J. Van, & Kapur, S. (2012). Seminar Schizophrenia. doi:10.1016/S0140-6736(09)60995-8enia. Lancet (London, England), 374(9690), 635–645. https://doi.org/10.1016/S0140-6736(09)60995-8

Pineda, O. L. (2017, January 31). Are sleep disorders associated with cognitive decline? Neurology, Vol. 88, p. e42. https://doi.org/10.1212/WNL.0000000000003601

Plum, F. (1972). Prospects for research on schizophrenia. 3. Neurophysiology. Neuropathological findings. Neurosciences Research Program Bulletin, 10(4), 384–388.

Raschetti, R., Albanese, E., Vanacore, N., & Maggini, M. (2007). Cholinesterase inhibitors in mild cognitive impairment: A systematic review of randomised trials. PLoS Medicine, 4(11), 1818–1828. https://doi.org/10.1371/journal.pmed.0040338

Rethinking personality disorder. (2015, February 21). The Lancet, 385(9969), 664. https://doi.org/10.1016/S0140-6736(15)60272-0

Rief, W., Burton, C., Frostholm, L., Henningsen, P., Kleinstäuber, M., Kop, W. J., ... van der Feltz-Cornelis, C. (2017). Core Outcome Domains for Clinical Trials on Somatic Symptom Disorder, Bodily Distress Disorder, and Functional Somatic Syndromes: European Network on Somatic Symptom Disorders Recommendations. Psychosomatic Medicine, 79(9), 1008–1015. https://doi.org/10.1097/PSY.0000000000000502

Roth, T. (2007, August 15). Insomnia: Definition, prevalence, etiology, and consequences. Journal of Clinical Sleep Medicine, Vol. 3.

Rush, A. J., Trivedi, M. H., Wisniewski, S. R., Nierenberg, A. A., Stewart, J. W., Warden, D., ... Fava, M. (2006). Acute and longer-term outcomes in depressed outpatients requiring one or several treatment steps: A STAR*D report. American Journal of Psychiatry, 163(11), 1905–1917. https://doi.org/10.1176/ajp.2006.163.11.1905

S Schneider, L. (2000). A critical review of cholinesterase inhibitors as a treatment modality in Alzheimer's disease. Dialogues in Clinical Neuroscience, 2(2), 111–128. Retrieved from http://www.ncbi.nlm.nih.gov/pubmed/22033801

Saah, T. (2005, June 29). The evolutionary origins and significance of drug addiction. Harm Reduction Journal, Vol. 2. https://doi.org/10.1186/1477-7517-2-8

Sadock, B. J., Sadock, V. A., & Sussman, N. (n.d.). Kaplan & Sadock's pocket handbook of psychiatric drug treatment.

Sadock, B., & Sadock, V. (2008). Kaplan & Sadock's concise textbook of clinical psychiatry. Retrieved from https://books.google.com/books?hl=en&lr=&id=ubG51n2NgfwC&oi=fnd&pg=PR7&dq=kaplan+and+sadocks&ots=to5B6rFgyY&sig=tuTkbRvHXt-v5cbTIcKRK-9ClFT4

Scanlon, D. (2013). Specific Learning Disability and Its Newest Definition: Which Is Comprehensive? and Which Is Insufficient? Journal of Learning Disabilities, 46(1), 26–33. https://doi.org/10.1177/0022219412464342

Schulte, E. E. (2015, November 1). Learning disorders: How pediatricians can help. Cleveland Clinic Journal of Medicine, Vol. 82, pp. S24–S28. https://doi.org/10.3949/ccjm.82.s1.05

Sharma, A., Sinha, K., & Vandenberg, B. (2017). Pricing as a means of controlling alcohol consumption. British Medical Bulletin, 123(1), 149–158. https://doi.org/10.1093/bmb/ldx020

Shear, M. K., Simon, N., Wall, M., Zisook, S., Neimeyer, R., Duan, N., ... Keshaviah, A. (2011). Complicated grief and related bereavement issues for DSM-5. Depression and Anxiety, 28(2), 103–117. https://doi.org/10.1002/da.20780

Shearin, E. N., & Linehan, M. M. (1994). Dialectical behavior therapy for borderline personality disorder: Theoretical and empirical foundations. Acta Psychiatrica Scandinavica, Supplement, 89(379), 61–68. https://doi.org/10.1111/j.1600-0447.1994.tb05820.x

Shohat-Ophir, G., Kaun, K. R., Azanchi, R., & Heberlein, U. (2012a). Sexual deprivation increases ethanol intake in Drosophila. Science, 335(6074), 1351–1355. https://doi.org/10.1126/science.1215932

Shohat-Ophir, G., Kaun, K. R., Azanchi, R., & Heberlein, U. (2012b). Sexual deprivation increases ethanol intake in Drosophila. Science, 335(6074), 1351–1355. https://doi.org/10.1126/science.1215932

Sinyor, M., Schaffer, A., & Levitt, A. (2010). The Sequenced Treatment Alternatives to Relieve Depression (STAR*D) trial: A review. Canadian Journal of Psychiatry, Vol. 55, pp. 126–135. https://doi.org/10.1177/070674371005500303

Sleep Disorders and Sleep Deprivation. (2006). In H. R. Colten & B. M. Altevogt (Eds.), Sleep Disorders and Sleep Deprivation. https://doi.org/10.17226/11617

Sng, A. A. H., & Janca, A. (2016). Mindfulness for personality disorders. Current Opinion in Psychiatry, Vol. 29, pp. 70–76. https://doi.org/10.1097/YCO.0000000000000213

Spiegel, D., Lewis-Fernández, R., Lanius, R., Vermetten, E., Simeon, D., & Friedman, M. (2013). Dissociative Disorders in DSM-5. Annual Review of Clinical Psychology, 9(1), 299–326. https://doi.org/10.1146/annurev-clinpsy-050212-185531

Thapar, A., Cooper, M., Eyre, O., & Langley, K. (2013, January). Practitioner review: What have we learnt about the causes of ADHD? Journal of Child Psychology and Psychiatry and Allied Disciplines, Vol. 54, pp. 3–16. https://doi.org/10.1111/j.1469-7610.2012.02611.x

Triebwasser, J., Chemerinski, E., Roussos, P., & Siever, L. J. (2013). Paranoid Personality Disorder. Journal of Personality Disorders, 27(6), 795–805. https://doi.org/10.1521/pedi_2012_26_055

Tyrer, P., Reed, G. M., & Crawford, M. J. (2015, February 21). Classification, assessment, prevalence, and effect of personality disorder. The Lancet, Vol. 385, pp. 717–726. https://doi.org/10.1016/S0140-6736(14)61995-4

Wang, B., Freeman, M. P., Nonacs, R., Viguera, A. C., & Cohen, L. S. (2010). Massachusetts General Hospital Handbook of General Hospital Psychiatry. In Massachusetts General Hospital Handbook of General Hospital Psychiatry. https://doi.org/10.1016/B978-1-4377-1927-7.00046-7

Weinbrecht, A., Schulze, L., Boettcher, J., & Renneberg, B. (2016, March 1). Avoidant Personality Disorder: a Current Review. Current Psychiatry Reports, Vol. 18, pp. 1–8. https://doi.org/10.1007/s11920-016-0665-6

Whiteford, H. A., Degenhardt, L., Rehm, J., Baxter, A. J., Ferrari, A. J., Erskine, H. E., ... Vos, T. (2013). Global burden of disease attributable to mental and substance use disorders: Findings from the Global Burden of Disease Study 2010. The Lancet, 382(9904), 1575–1586. https://doi.org/10.1016/S0140-6736(13)61611-6

Widiger, T. A. (2015). Assessment of DSM-5 Personality Disorder. Journal of Personality Assessment, 97(5), 456–466. https://doi.org/10.1080/00223891.2015.1041142

Yaribeygi, H., Panahi, Y., Sahraei, H., Johnston, T. P., & Sahebkar, A. (2017, July 21). The impact of stress on body function: A review. EXCLI Journal, Vol. 16, pp. 1057–1072. https://doi.org/10.17179/excli2017-480

Yatham, L. N., Kennedy, S. H., Parikh, S. v., Schaffer, A., Bond, D. J., Frey, B. N., ... Berk, M. (2018). Canadian Network for Mood and Anxiety Treatments (CANMAT) and International Society for Bipolar Disorders (ISBD) 2018 guidelines for the management of patients with bipolar disorder. Bipolar Disorders, 20(2), 97–170. https://doi.org/10.1111/bdi.12609

Yehuda, R. (2002). Current Concepts: Post-Traumtic Stress Disorder. The New England Journal of Medicine, 346(2), 108–114. https://doi.org/10.1056/NEJMra012941

Youssef, N. A., Ege, M., Angly, S. S., Strauss, J. L., & Marx, C. E. (2011). Is obstructive sleep apnea associated with ADHD? Annals of Clinical Psychiatry : Official Journal of the American Academy of Clinical Psychiatrists, 23(3), 213–224. Retrieved from http://www.ncbi.nlm.nih.gov/pubmed/21808754

Yuen, K. M., & Pelayo, R. (2017a). Socioeconomic Impact of Pediatric Sleep Disorders. Sleep Medicine Clinics, 12(1), 23–30. https://doi.org/10.1016/j.jsmc.2016.10.005

Yuen, K. M., & Pelayo, R. (2017b, March 1). Socioeconomic Impact of Pediatric Sleep Disorders. Sleep Medicine Clinics, Vol. 12, pp. 23–30. https://doi.org/10.1016/j.jsmc.2016.10.005

Zipfel, S., Giel, K. E., Bulik, C. M., Hay, P., & Schmidt, U. (2015). Anorexia nervosa: aetiology, assessment, and treatment. The Lancet. Psychiatry, 2(12), 1099–1111. https://doi.org/10.1016/S2215-0366(15)00356-9

Index

A

Acute Dystonia 197
Acute stress disorder 79
ADHD 147
Adjustment Disorder 80
Adrenaline 24
Agoraphobia 59
Akathisia 198
amygdala 22
Antidepressants 200
  Treatment of Anxiety 68
Antipsychotics 193
Anxiety 54
Anxiolytics 69, 212
asylum movement 8
Attention Deficit/Hyperactivity Disorder 147
Augmentation of antidepressants 44
Autism spectrum disorders
  OCD 65
Autism Spectrum Disorders (ASD) 143
Aversion therapy 219

B

Bedlam 7
Behavior Therapy 218
Bipolar depression 47
Bipolar Disorder 45
Bleuler, Eugen 10
Body Focused Repetitive Behaviors
  OCD 67
Brain 17
brain stem 22
Bruxism 177

C

Carbamazepine 210
Cataplexy 173
Catatonia 33
Causes, of schizophrenia 29
CBT for insomnia (CBTi) 170
Charcot 8
Charcot, Jean-Martin 8
Chief Complaint 222
Childhood-Onset Fluency Disorder 159
Choosing an Antidepressant 201
Circadian Rhythm Sleep Disorders 175
Cognitive Behavioral Therapy 216
Cognitive Therapy 217
Communication Disorders 158
Compulsions 64
Compulsive Shopping 165
Concrete Operational Stage 14
Conduct Disorder 164
Confusing Things About Bipolar Disorder 51
Coprophilia 191
Cortex 21
Crisis Intervention 215

D

Delayed Ejaculation , 183
Delirium 27
Delusion 32
Dementia 135
Depression and chronic pain 40
Depression in other illnesses 41
Descartes 6
Developmental Coordination Disorder 155
Dialectical Behavior Therapy 219
Discontinuation Syndrome 203
Disruptive Mood Dysregulation Disorder 163
Dopamine 24, 178
Dual-sex therapy 185
Dual-sex Therapy 185

Duchenne 8
Dysthymia 40

E

Electroconvulsive Therapy (ECT) 44
Elimination Disorders 160
Encopresis 162
Endocannabinoids 25
Endorphins 25
Enuresis 161
EPS 197
Erectile Disorder , 182
Exhibitionism , 190
Extra Pyramidal Symptoms 197

F

Female Orgasmic Disorder , 183
Female Sexual Interest/Arousal Disorder , 182
Fetishism , 190
Formal Operational Stage 14
Frotteurism , 190

G

GABA 24
Gender dysphoria 188
Gender Dysphoria 188
Generalized anxiety disorder 55
Genito-pelvic Pain/Penetration Disorder , 184
Glutamate 24
Group Therapy 216

H

Hallucinations 31
Happiness 228
Hippocrates 5
Histamine 24
Hoarding 67
Human Development 13
Human Sexuality 178
Hypersomnolence Disorder 172

hypothalamus 22

I

Inner Brain 22
Insight 33
Intellectual Disabilities 152
Intermittent Explosive Disorder 164
Internet Addiction 165

K

Keshavan 36
Kleptomania 164
Klismaphilia 191

L

Lamotrigine 211
Language Disorder 160
Learning Theory 12
Lithium Carbonate 209

M

Major Depressive Disorder 38
Male Hypoactive Sexual Disorder , 182
Mania 47
MAOI 204
Medical Marijuana 230
Medications Used in Sex Therapy 186
Melancholy 5
Mental status examination 225
Metabolic Syndrome 199
Monoamine Oxidase Inhibitors (MAOIs) 204
Mood Stabilizers 207
Motor Disorders 155

N

Narcolepsy 173
Nature vs. Nurture 227
Necrophilia , 191

Negative Symptoms 33
Neurasthenia 9
Neuroleptic Malignant Syndrome 200
Neuron 17
Neurotransmitters 23
Normal Sleep 166
NREM Sleep 167

O

Obsessions 63
Obsessive-Compulsive Disorder (OCD) 62
Obsessive Compulsive Personality Disorder or OCPD
OCD 65
Open-ended 222
Operant conditioning 13
Oppositional Defiant Disorder 162
Other Antidepressants 205
Oxcarbazepine 212
Oxytocin 25, 179

P

PANDAS 66
Panic Disorder 56
Paraphilias , 189
Parasomnias 176
Parasomnias Associated with REM Sleep 176
Parkinsonism 198
PDE5 inhibitors 186
Persistent Complex Bereavement Disorder 80
Phentolamine 186
Postpartum depression 41
Premature Ejaculation , 183
Premenstrual Dysphoric Disorder (PMDD) 41
Psychiatric Evaluation 223
Psychoanalysis 14, 214
Psychoanalytic Psychotherapy 215
Psychosis and bipolar 52

Psychotherapy 214
PTSD 75
Pussin, Jean-Baptiste 7
Pyromania 165

Q

QT Prolongation 199

R

Rapport 221
REM Sleep 167

S

Schizoaffective disorder 36
Schizophrenia 28
Selective Serotonin Reuptake Inhibitors 201
Separation Anxiety Disorder 61
Serotonin 24
Serotonin Norepinephrine Reuptake Inhibitors 203
Serotonin syndrome 202
Sex Addiction 187
Sexual masochism , 190
Sexual sadism , 190
Sleep 166
Sleep Apnea 173
Sleep Disorders 170
Sleep Hygiene 169
SNRI 203
Social Anxiety Disorder (Social Phobia) 60
Social (Pragmatic) Communication Disorder 160
Specific Learning Disorders 157
Specific Phobias 61
Speech Sound Disorder 158
SSRIs 201
STAR*D 45
Stereotypic Movement Disorder 156
Stuttering 159
Substance/Medication induced Sexu-

al Dysfunction , 184
Synapse 18

T

thalamus 22
Thought Disorder 32
Tic Disorders 156
Transvestism , 191
Trauma 75
Treatment
  PTSD 78
Treatment of Anxiety disorders 68
Treatment of MDD 42
Treatment, of schizophrenia 34
Treatment of Sexual Dysfunction 185
Tricyclic Antidepressants 203

V

Valproic Acid 210
Vedas 5
Video Game Addiction 165
Voyeurism , 190

W

Wernicke, Carl 8

Z

Zeitgebers 175
Zoophilia , 191

Ten things you don't know
About the Author

1. In high school, he very "mysteriously" developed a fever the day before he was supposed to go to a military-style camp.
2. The fever "mysteriously" disappeared when he was told to skip the camp and go on vacation with the family.
3. As a medical student, in his first lecture of psychiatry, when the professor started his lecture with "Mental illness is divided into two types…," he murmured from the last bench, "Curable and incurable."
4. Again, as a medical student, when a hapless professor asked the rhetorical question in the class "Does anyone know what marriage counseling is?" he responded, "It is a discussion of what to do, when to do and how to do." The professor was not amused and reprimanded him for unprofessional behavior.
5. He developed a mysterious illness while visiting a beloved friend Dr. JPD, who was sick in the hospital. He mysteriously got sick and felt a compelling need to get inside the sheets as he suddenly felt very cold. As this happened in the presence of a dozen esteemed psychiatrists, it was quickly deemed as an attention-seeking stunt, and he was diagnosed with a conversion disorder.
6. The same attention-seeking stunt happened again when he was alone. He wondered how he could try to "trick" himself, or try to get his own attention, and feared that his case of conversion might be very severe or "incurable." A few days later, he was promptly diagnosed with malaria and was treated appropriately - which ended the conversion disorder, but not his attention-seeking behavior.
7. As a trainee, in the presence of a psychoanalyst who was advising the trainees to get therapy by saying, "If you are going to provide therapy, you should undergo therapy." He quipped "I am glad I am not learning obstetrics." Again, the professor was not amused.
8. He has a reputation for not giving what the patient wants, and in one of the clinics where he worked, he set a record for patient complaints.
9. He continued to set a similar record in his next job.
10. So, he decided to write this book.

www.ingramcontent.com/pod-product-compliance
Lightning Source LLC
Chambersburg PA
CBHW030613220526
45463CB00004B/1283